ENDURING CANCER

CRITICAL GLOBAL HEALTH   Evidence, Efficacy, Ethnography
A series edited by Vincanne Adams and João Biehl

ENDURING CANCER

LIFE, DEATH, AND

DWAIPAYAN BANERJEE

DIAGNOSIS IN DELHI

Duke University Press *Durham and London* 2020

© 2020 DUKE UNIVERSITY PRESS. All rights reserved
Designed by Courtney Leigh Richardson. Typeset in Minion Pro
and Fengardo Neue by Copperline Book Services.
Library of Congress Cataloging-in-Publication Data
Names: Banerjee, Dwaipayan, [date] author.
Title: Enduring cancer : life, death, and diagnosis in Delhi /
Dwaipayan Banerjee.
Other titles: Critical global health.
Description: Durham : Duke University Press, 2020. |
Series: Critical global health | Includes bibliographical references
and index.
Identifiers: LCCN 2019050711 (print)
LCCN 2019050712 (ebook)
ISBN 9781478008620 (hardcover)
ISBN 9781478009559 (paperback)
ISBN 9781478012214 (ebook)
Subjects: LCSH: Cancer—Treatment—India—Delhi. |
Cancer—Diagnosis—Social aspects—India. | Cancer—
Diagnosis—India—Psychological aspects. | Poor—India— Delhi—
Social conditions—21st century.
Classification: LCC RA645. C3 B36 2020 (print) |
LCC RA645. C3 (ebook) | DDC 616.99/4—dc23
LC record available at https://lccn.loc.gov/2019050711
LC ebook record available at https://lccn.loc.gov/2019050712

COVER ART: Bird
clinic, Delhi, India,
1985. Photo by Carl De
Keyzer. Courtesy of Carl
De Keyzer/Magnum
Photos.

CONTENTS

ACKNOWLEDGMENTS

This book's debts are innumerable and run deep. I began my anthropological career as a graduate student at the Delhi School of Economics and only continued thanks to my inspirational teachers there. My adviser Deepak Mehta introduced me to a world of ideas and the joys of transgressing disciplinary boundaries, while Rita Brara taught me the value of reading closely and not just between the lines. Rajni Palriwala and Meenakshi Thapan's mentorship gave me the confidence to venture further, as did the many conversations in and outside the canteen with other teachers and friends. I was fortunate to have my doctoral training continue at New York University with Emily Martin and Tejaswini Ganti. Emily's work as well as her guidance of mine have been a model of thought and care. Her critical support through the many twists and turns of my research is the reason this book has come to fruition. Teja taught me not only to think clearly but also what it means to live and breathe one's research. Without Rayna Rapp's infinite patience, I would not have dared venture into medical anthropology late into graduate school; every page of this book is imprinted with her training. Her patience was only matched by that of Faye Ginsburg, who read and transformed many drafts of chapters and proposals. Helena Hansen's guidance at the final stage of this book's first draft was invaluable in clarifying its argument. At the New School, a few streets north of my academic home, Ann Stoler's remarkable pedagogy reminded me that thinking and writing could be exciting. I only hope that my work reflects the quality of the engagement of such remarkable mentors.

Thanks to my many other wonderful senior colleagues at NYU, including Aisha Khan, Allen Feldman, Andrew Romig, Angela Zito, Ara Merjian, Bambi Schieffelin, Bruce Grant, Cheryl Furjanic, Fred Myers, Gwynneth Malin, Jane Tylus, Melissa Burtt, Noelle Stout, Sally Merry, Susan Murray, Thomas Looser, and Zeb Tortorici. Thanks also to my NYU friends: Ademide Adelusi-Adeluyi, Alison Cool, Alyse Takayesu, Amali Ibrahim,

Amy Lasater-Wille, Brinton Ahlin, Cara Shousterman, Catalina Arango, Dania Hückmann, Delia Solomons, Eduardo Matos-Martín, Emily Cohen, Emily Yates-Doerr, Ernesto de Carvalho, Eugenia Kisin, Grace Gu, Hyejin Nah, Irina Levin, JM DeLeon, Johanna Römer, Lee Douglas, Lily Defriend, Louis Römer, Narges Bajoghli, Natasha Raheja, Rachel Lears, Ram Natarajan, Robert Chang, Sandra Rozental, Schuyler Marquez, Tate LeFevre, Teresa Montoya, Tiana Hayden, Tyler Zoanni, Vanessa Agard-Jones, Vibhuti Ramachandran, Vijayanka Nair, Wenrui Chen, Will Thomson, Yasmin Moll, and Jennifer Heuson. When I was a postdoctoral fellow at Dartmouth College, Sienna Craig was an exemplary early-career mentor, whose model of teaching and writing I aspire to emulate. The writing workshop Sienna runs with Laura Ogden is a uniquely supportive academic space; thanks to Yana Stainova and Chelsey Kivland, among others, who helped craft some of the passages that appear in this text. Thanks also to Dale Eickelman, Deborah Nichols, Doug Haynes, Elizabeth Carpenter-Song, John Watanabe, Sergei Kan, and William Elison for your Hanover warmth.

Over the last three years, my home at the MIT Program for Science, Technology and Society has been more than kind in allowing me the time and resources to finish this project. My thanks to my wonderful colleagues Amy Moran-Thomas, Beth Semel, Caley Horan, Carolyn Carlson, Christine Walley, David Mindell, Deborah Fitzgerald, Eden Medina, Erica James, Graham Jones, Gus Zahariadis, Harriet Ritvo, Heather Paxson, John Durant, Judith Spitzer, Karen Gardner, Kate Brown, Kenneth Manning, Merritt Roe Smith, Paree Pinkney, Robin Scheffler, Rosalind Williams, Sana Aiyar, Sherry Turkle, Tanalis Padilla, and William Deringer. In particular, the program allowed me to convene a book workshop whose conversations have fundamentally shaped the chapters that follow. Carlo Caduff, Harris Solomon, Michael Fischer, and Sarah Pinto, you will not miss your deep impress on this text; thank you for your generosity over that day and since. Clapperton Mavhunga, David Kaiser, Jennifer Light, and Stefan Helmreich, a special thanks for your generous mentorship.

Over the years, I have learned in many intangible ways from scholars across many universities and contexts. Each of you, in your own way, has made this text possible: Aditi Malik, Aditya Sarkar, Ajay Skaria, Alex Nading, Aliya Rao, Amen Jaffer, Amit Prasad, Amy Krauss, Ana Maria Ulloa, Anand Vaidya, Anand Taneja, Andrew Brandel, Ashawari Chaudhari, Banu Subramaniam, Benjamin Siegel, Bharat Venkat, Bhrigupati Singh, Cecilia Van Hollen, Chandan Bose, Clara Han, Cori Hayden, Danielle Carr, Darja

Djordjevic, David Jones, David Macdougall, Divya Cherian, Durba Mitra, Eram Alam, Gabriela Soto Laveaga, Hemangini Gupta, Janelle Lamoreaux, Juliet McMullin, Karen-Sue Taussig, Kartik Nair, Katie Detwiler, Katyayani Dalmia, Kiran Kumbhar, Lan Li, Lawrence Liang, Lilly Irani, Lucas Mueller, Marissa Mika, Martin Lin, Maya Ratnam, Maura Finkelstein, Megan Moodie-Brasoveanu, Megha Sehdev, Miryam Nacimento, Namrata Ghosh, Nicolas Langlitz, Nishita Trisal, Nivedita Ghosh, Poulami Roychowdhury, Prakash Kumar, Projit Mukharji, Puneet Bhasin, Radhika Govindrajan, Rohit De, Saiba Varma, Sandra Bärnreuther, Sarah Besky, Sareeta Amrute, Sophia Powers, Subhadeepta Ray, Sunayana Ganguly, Swayam Bagaria, Tamara Fernandez, Tulasi Srinivas, Vaibhav Saria, Vincanne Adams, and Zoë Wool. Aditi Saraf, we have endured for almost two decades; this is now for keeps. Moyukh Chatterjee, the phone bills speak for themselves. Thanks to Sandipto Dasgupta, for being an exemplary scholar-housemate, in most ways. And Debashree Mukherjee, writing companion extraordinaire, thank you. Families come in many forms. To my Boston family—Kareem Khubchandani, Gowri Vijayakumar, and Josh Williams—aunties of the world really do unite. Ishani Saraf and William Stafford, for being oases of sanity across so many academic venues. Jacob Copeman, I am disbelieving that we managed to coauthor a book without ever being on the same continent; I still need proof that you are real. My Delhi friends and elders, a special thank you: Amba-Suhasini Jhala, Anirudh Nair, Babli and Kanti Saraf, Isheeta Mustafi, Priyanka Pruthi, Raghu Karnad, and Sumit Roy. In the United States, for supporting me in a new environment, thank you to Abigail Savitch-Lew, Anthony Miler, Brandon Hamilton, David Powers, Hande Inanc, Harsher Singh, Ishita Srivastava, Jeffrey Lenowitz, Jyothi Natarajan, Max Powers, Nada Jung, Sally Powers, Sarah Fajardo, Shruti Ravindran, and Uma Anand. Kerry (and Bodhi) Jessup; I owe you more than I can put into words here. Thanks to my parents for trusting in me enough as I took the jump into academia. My family—the Banerjee and Datta clans—you have been an inspiration since my earliest memories. Rat, my cat, thank you for allowing me to write while you napped.

I would be remiss not to mention a few books that have fundamentally shaped my writing here: they include *Life and Words*; *Affliction*; *Improvising Medicine*; *Malignant*; *Where There Is No Midwife*; *Daughters of Parvati*; and *No Aging in India*. Veena Das, Sarah Pinto, Lochlann Jain, and Lawrence Cohen, it has been a privilege to be allowed into your thoughts, and I look forward to continuing to learn from you. Kavita Sivaramakrishnan, your work gave me insight into this project in a way only you can really understand.

The research for this book was made possible by the support of a McCracken Fellowship at NYU and fellowships from the Wenner-Gren Foundation, the National Science Foundation, the Humanities Initiative at NYU, and a Mellon postdoctoral fellowship at the Leslie Center for the Humanities and the Department of Anthropology at Dartmouth College. Molly Mullin, you were the first reader of this text; thank you for your painstaking editing. Thank you, Kenneth Wissoker, for seeing the promise of this book and for the effortless way in which you brought it into being. You found readers whose attentiveness was beyond my expectations. They have so deeply shaped the book that they deserve all the credit (and none of the blame) for the pages that follow. Thank you also, Joshua Tranen, for your editorial labor in producing these pages.

Finally, this book is dedicated to the tireless cancer care workers in Delhi—doctors, nurses, counselors, and NGO staff—who welcomed me into their world and work. I refrain from naming them here to preserve their anonymity. While I have taken the liberty of writing about your efforts with a measure of academic distance, I remain in awe of your tireless capacities for care.

INTRODUCTION

I

I am at a messy table, full of government forms, medical instruments, and diagnostic charts. Across me, Sameera, a young medical resident, has just finished attending to about eighty patients in less than three hours. We are at the cancer ward of one of India's largest, busiest, and best-regarded public hospitals—the All India Institute of the Medical Sciences (AIIMS). Cancer patients flock here by the thousands from all over the country. Many know that if the long journey here does not push their disease past the possibility of treatment, the months-long wait times once they reach AIIMS will. At this moment, in the early days of my fieldwork, I am confused about how the word "cancer" is never spoken. I have already seen how many patients are not told their diagnosis even until their death, and how families often react with anger upon hearing the word. In India's largest cancer ward, nobody seems to have cancer.

I know about a reticence in speaking about the disease in many parts of the world, but I am interested in finding out why it is particularly pronounced here. If patients do not know they have cancer, I ask Sameera, what brings them to an oncology ward for treatment? Exhausted, she looks up and says elliptically: *shak*. The Hindi word *shak* is translatable as "doubt," "skepticism," or "suspicion." Unsure of what she means, I continue to push her. If *shak* first brings patients to the clinic, why is it not dealt with, why do you not tell them what they have, how long they will live? Putting her pen down, she elaborates. "You see, shak does not just mean they are unsure about what disease they have. It also means they do not know whether they will be able to afford treatment, whether their family or neighbors will stand by them. Later, shak will stand between us doctors and them, whether they trust us when we advise a lengthy treatment, or when we tell them that there is nothing more to do."

I have just traveled with a Delhi cancer care nongovernmental organization (NGO) during their home visit to a patient who lives in the outskirts of the city. Our car had broken down earlier, and we traveled the last miles in the official NGO van with its logo "Caring for Cancer" printed on the door. The patient—Amarjit—was a man in his seventies. Amarjit seemed visibly discomfited by the logo: he absolutely did not have cancer, he asserted. In his refusal to name his diagnosis, he was exemplary of many others who resisted the enclosure of his disease within an already fixed script. The nurse expertly played along, hoping to transact care on his terms rather than her own. She asked, "Aapke khyala mein aapko kya hua hain?" (What do you think has happened to you?). The Hindi word *khyala* translates to "thought" as well as "care." His careful reply was that he had "oncology," a dexterous negotiation of the word "cancer" and all that the diagnosis entailed.

Accompanying a different team from the same NGO a few weeks later, I visited a young couple, Malika and Madanlal. Malika had recently been diagnosed with breast cancer. As I walked in, I was struck by how different their one-room home was from others I had seen in the neighborhood: it was beautifully painted, and ornate new moldings lined the walls and window. Later, the NGO workers told me that Malika had been in pain and depressed after her diagnosis. While she was hospitalized, Madanlal, a construction worker, had borrowed money and materials from his employer and remade their room. He had crafted it with Malika's favorite designs and colors and covered the walls with framed photos from when they had vacationed as newlyweds. To ameliorate her pain, Madanlal had taken it upon himself to literally rebuild Malika's collapsing world.

These fragments offer a glimpse into the concern of this book: the efforts of patients, families, physicians, and cancer care workers in Delhi to manage the unsettling force of a cancer diagnosis. With a word, *shak*, Sameera described the power of the disease and the disrupted social relations it left in its wake. With a word, she synopsized a feeling that recurs in the narratives of cancer patients all over the world—a sense of being unmoored from prior certainties about oneself and one's place in the world. When cancer appears, it distributes itself across networks of social relations, testing them for strength and vulnerability. In Madanlal and Malika's case the ties between them proved resilient, helping mitigate the shock and force of the diagnosis. In time Malika would recover, bolstered in part by the efforts of her kin to sustain the world in which she lived. But often, the diagnosis put pressure on already fragile social bonds, pushing capacities of endurance to the point of their exhaustion. Many, like Amarjit, chose to conceal their cancer because they did not trust the worlds in which they lived to welcome them.

To live with cancer in Delhi, then, was to navigate the many doubts, suspicions, and skepticisms that spread through social relations in the wake of a cancer diagnosis. Those who lived with or alongside the disease had to account for which medical institutions and practitioners were affordable and dependable, which neighbors and kin they could trust and who might wish them harm, and whether old histories of violence and resentment within marriages would resurface in this time of vulnerability. In these and many other ways, to live with cancer, my interlocutors had to figure out more than the capacity of bodies to withstand and respond to therapies. They also had to learn the strengths and vulnerabilities of the social worlds within which the disease unfolded, the kinds of speech and action that would be conducive to their well-being, and the infrastructures of care and neglect that would shape the trajectory of their treatments. In this book, I present the efforts of my interlocutors to live within these shifting tensilities of social relations in the wake of cancer. I argue that living with and alongside the disease was to be newly awakened to the fragility of social ties, some already made brittle by past histories, and others that would be retested for their capacity to support.

Such an attunement to the fragility of social relations around cancer helps me explain how the disease is experienced in a specific place and time. While investigating the force and impact of a cancer diagnosis upon social relations, I found older cracks and fault lines: long-standing failures in Indian medical care, prior betrayals in marriages, and personal histories that made some more vulnerable to the consequences of the disease. For example, this ethnography unfolds in Delhi, where for most of the urban poor a cancer diagnosis came too late for curative intervention. That is, long wait times in public health facilities ensured that the disease would have progressed beyond the time of cancer's traditional treatment modalities: chemotherapy, surgery, and radiation. Often, then, when cancer appeared in con-

ditions of long-standing precarity, the disease articulated with past vulnerabilities, inflecting their points of stress in new and urgent ways. A cancer
diagnosis was the latest and most serious in a long series of infrastructural,
domestic, and familial episodes of failure and violence. My effort in this
book is to present a picture of how cancer settled into these longer histories
of vulnerability, and how these forces of the past shaped the contours of life
around and after diagnosis.

Thinking about such an accretive impact of a cancer diagnosis—as it articulates past vulnerabilities with new pressures—goes against the grain of
how it is often represented: as a cataclysmic breakdown of a person's social
world, inaugurating a new life in the "kingdom of the sick" (to paraphrase
Susan Sontag).[1] Without discounting the dramatic impact of the disease's
diagnosis, my aim is to supplement such accounts of rupture with one of
continuities, tracing how a person's past reverberated into his or her present and future. To understand the continuities between a pre- and post-
diagnosed self is to understand how the disease sedimented into the give-
and-take of everyday life, rather than marking a departure from it. It is to
understand, for example, how the disease nestled into or tore apart already
fragile kinship ties, why my interlocutors spoke indirectly or not at all about
the disease to those closest to them, and why some within the same neighborhoods could access treatment while others could not. Thinking of the
impact of cancer in such an accretive way helps uncover the long durability
of social doubts in everyday life within which the disease took shape, not
rupturing prior certainties, but inflecting long-standing vulnerabilities in
new and subtle ways.

The chapters that follow build on this underlying insight: when cancer
appeared in conditions of precarity, it put further pressure on already frayed
social relations; living with cancer entailed living with a pervasive doubt
about the viability of such relations. In this space, my interlocutors experimented with strategies to negotiate this doubt, never entirely dispelling it,
but keeping its capacity to overwhelm at bay. In such circumstances, the diagnosis of cancer cannot be described as a critical breakdown in an otherwise stable life, because in conditions of precarity, such certainties about
one's health and well-being were never easily at hand. The concern of this
book, then, is to describe such experiments to live with or alongside cancer, managing doubts about social relations in *already* fragile worlds. In the
book's concluding chapter, I understand these experiments in relations as
demonstrative of an ethics of endurance. Suspicions and deficits of trust
never came to be entirely dispelled or absorbed by the strategies invented

to manage them. This was not only because treatments were often scarce or because remission was always a risk, but also because efforts to maintain brittle social ties around a patient required continuous work. The analytic of endurance aims to explain this durability of doubt—in bodies, social relations, and institutions—that remained ever-present, guiding what it meant to live with or alongside cancer.

More specifically, I thematize these experiments with doubt and social relations across three fields: a circumspection of speech about the disease, the problem of cancer pain, and the dangers and possibilities of its aesthetic representation. Across each of these fields, I describe strategies to manage doubts about social relations awakened by cancer diagnoses. For example, concealing diagnoses was often a strategy through which my interlocutors anticipated how their pasts would reverberate into the future: telling some and not others helped them maintain a sense of continuity in their lives, as well as guard against those whom they already mistrusted. The problem of cancer pain similarly required a testing of fragile social ties. In a context where diagnosis often came too late, the physical pain that accompanied cancer became more than a "side effect," pushing public health workers to take it on as a central concern. In investigating this prominence of pain in Indian cancer care, I show how its meaning (as a research subject) and amelioration (as a therapeutic practice) depended on apprehending the fragility of a patient's social world. Finally, in exploring aesthetic accounts of cancer in India (primarily in films and memoirs), I examine attempts parallel to my own to investigate the disease's social reverberations. Many of these aesthetic accounts are pedagogical, offering moral lessons about how to correctly respond to the disease and, in the process, establish a proper national, gendered, and psychological state. Other accounts reject such transformative visions, exploring the durable consequences of the disease that could not be so easily transcended. In describing these contrasting moral visions, I explain the dangers of aesthetic abstractions that erase cancer's everyday stakes while also exploring the felicity of those that do not. In the process, I sharpen my own ethnographic sense of the fraught socialities that cohere around the disease.

Concealing Cancer

Amarjit's response—that he really had "oncology" and not cancer—was one way, among others, through which my fieldwork interlocutors evaded directly naming the diagnosis. This tricky relationship between language and cancer continuously haunted my fieldwork, never quite resolving itself. Looking through more than six hundred patient records at AIIMS, I found that more than 80 percent of the patients had been recorded as being "unaware" of their diagnosis when they came to the clinic. But, through the course of my research, I came to understand the limits of the word "unaware." Patients and families often came to the ward and hid prognoses they had received from other doctors or oncologists. At other times, they colluded to conceal their diagnosis from neighbors and kin. And most frequently, family members colluded with each other to protect patients from the perceived psychic impact of the word. In these cases, patients were almost always more "aware" of their disease than family members imagined them to be. Throughout my fieldwork, I would find their motivations for concealment as varied as the practices through which secrets were sustained.

Yet, despite this variance in motivations and practice, I understand concealment as part of a broader repertoire of strategies to apprehend and mitigate fragile social relations put under pressure by cancer. For example, by hiding prior diagnoses from new doctors, some patients and families evidenced their skepticism about biomedical practitioners and institutions. Many believed that revealing a bleak prognosis to a new physician would hurt their chances of accessing care. In such instances, concealment was indicative not of a hope of recovery but of a deep deficit of trust between poorer patients and medical institutions. However, while I describe a few moments of diagnostic nondisclosure, the forms of concealment I pay most attention to are those that unfolded *after* diagnosis, in the homes of patients and among kin, neighbors, and NGO caregivers. I do this in keeping with my effort throughout the book to pay attention to the slow reverberations of cancer, shifting attention away from the life-altering moment of diagnosis that preoccupies the sociomedical literature concerned with the disease. In these homes, intimate and neighborly relations were often already undermined by past histories of violence or neglect. When cancer care NGO workers entered these fraught worlds to offer care, they understood that they would need to work on reknitting these frayed relational threads. Often, this meant maintaining fictions of concealment. Working alongside these cancer care workers, who were ethnographers in their own right, I came to understand how negotiating the vulnerabilities around cancer involved deciding whether, when, and how much to reveal about diagnoses. Over time, patients, families, and palliative care workers would experiment with these relations, testing what could be said without incurring harm. For example, for one young cancer patient, concealment became a way of safeguarding his livelihood. He earned his small income by running errands for his neighbors and believed that revealing his diagnosis would isolate him, taking away the money he required for treatment. For many others, concealing became a way to avoid the psychic damage caused by well-meaning kin and neighbors who would often begin mourning living patients as if they were already dead. And for still others, concealing became a way to maintain the hope of a future together, even while knowing full well that such optimism was unwarranted.

More broadly, I argue that such practices of concealment evidence a pervasive subjunctive mood in the experience of cancer in Delhi. As anthropologists understand it, the subjunctive mood is a world ordered through narrative or rituals *as if* it were real, but separate from lived reality.[2] They are illusions that are not intended as lies, but rather as a play with another possible reality, a mutual entry into the worlds of "could be," when the "is" might have become too difficult to bear. While judgments based on sincerity and authenticity might find such illusory plays difficult to accept, they are crucial to all kinds of social rituals, expressing possibilities rather than actualities.[3] Often, the conjuring up of the subjunctive reflects that ordinary life has become so overwhelming that the subjunctive mood allows for another, incongruous world. I present this explanation of the subjunctive because it captures the relation between the lived experience of cancer and the active concealments of its diagnosis. Social rituals of concealment opened the possibility of another world in which cancer did not shape and deform every moment of social life. Thinking about the subjunctive mood in contexts of illness, Byron and Mary-Jo DelVecchio Good and Veena Das separately describe it as allowing for traffic in human possibilities rather than certainties, keeping alive multiple perspectives, emotions, and moods as a way to cope with the harms of disease.[4] Developing this insight, I describe concealment as a practice of inhabiting the subjunctive mood, as patients, kin, caregivers, and physicians helped sustain possibilities of relations that disclosures might foreclose.

Importantly, in anthropological description of rituals as worlds of the subjunctive, the "other worlds" that rituals create are not escapist fantasies, but rather a realist assessment that this world cannot always be bent to one's will.[5] In consonance, I stress that in concealing their diagnosis, my interlocutors were not escaping or denying the truth and consequences of cancer. They did not misunderstand its force or believe that by simply not speaking about their disease, it would go away. I argue to the contrary that by concealing, they opened a range of reflections on the actual circumstances of their lives. To not name the disease was often a tacit expression of a knowledge of infrastructural failure: What use was speech when treatments were not easily at hand, or had not been at the appropriate time? At other times, concealment could indicate the presence of untrustworthy kin or neighbors. And in yet other instances, it was often a sign of care and thoughtfulness. Taken together, these practices of concealment shared one feature: they reflected on the intransigent social circumstances within which the disease appeared.

Pointing out that practices of concealment are not escapist is important because, as Cecilia Van Hollen describes in her work, biomedical ethicists and public health researchers have made them out to be so.[6] Such bioethical discourses, committed to autonomy and transparency, understand any prevarication about revealing diagnoses as evidence of medical noncompliance or as a contravention of the patient's right to know. But as Byron and Mary-Jo DelVecchio Good as well as Van Hollen show, even when cancer bioethics seem universal and ahistorical, the norm that diagnoses must always be disclosed is one of fairly recent vintage.[7] Further, in practice, such norms are often a red herring, when ethical decision making in the real world has little to do with the abstract principles that are supposed to guide them.[8] The practices of concealment I describe reveal biomedical ethics in practice, from the point of view of those who experience their disease and navigate its consequences in their everyday lives.

Further, writing about medical nondisclosure in the context of pregnancy in rural India, Sarah Pinto describes the biomedical imperative of transparency as casting social worlds into distinct domains of compliance and noncompliance, rationality and irrationality.[9] Within this context, Pinto explains how the near-silences of pregnant women are often misrecognized by doctors and NGOs as perversely normalizing the pathological fact of infant death, as evidence of a putatively Indian propensity toward fatalism, or as plain rural ignorance about health. Similarly, I describe how the medical literature on cancer in India consistently misreads practices of concealment as evidence of an "Indian" capacity to accept and reconcile with the inevitability of loss. Some describe this acceptance as fatalism, while others call it denial; some encourage its mobilization in the clinical encounter to bolster coping, while others castigate it as ignorance of the truth of cancer. Resisting such readings of acts of concealment as evidence of lack, I show instead that they reveal ethical negotiations with already fraught circumstances. As Pinto too recognized in her work, acts of concealment did not "normalize" difficult circumstances, but rather revealed how encounters with life-threatening suffering haunted already fragile worlds.

As such, my understanding of the stakes of concealment departs from bioethics and comes closest to Anne-Lise François's description of an ethics of "recessive action."[10] François thinks of concealment as more than just the absence of knowledge and transparency. Instead, she understands concealment as a release from the imperative of actions that knowledge often demands. I share François's refusal of the equation of action with agency and concealment with passivity. Rather, I argue that concealment reveals an ethical way of being, not circumscribed to the meaning of ethics as acting upon the world to better oneself. It reveals the capacity to *not* act in the face of knowledge and of the potentially destructive consequences of action. In the following, I show that concealment sometimes evidences an ethics of responsiveness to conditions where revelation holds danger. These are acts of ordinary ethics, grown from within preexisting economies of speech and silence.[11] I argue, then, that describing concealment as denial or escapism is exactly the wrong way to understand its practice in the lives of the urban poor in Delhi. Instead, "escapist" better describes the hubris of public health dogma that believes disclosure and transparency are necessary preconditions for better health.

Cancer Becomes Pain

Pain has long been theorized as a condition so ensconced in doubt that it poses a biological limit to sociality. For example, Elaine Scarry's canonical description of pain stresses its capacity to destroy language, causing a reversion to "the pre-language of cries."[12] Scarry reserves for pain a unique ontological status, thinking it capable of producing a doubt in relations so intense that it creates an unbridgeable chasm between the person who witnesses and the one who suffers. Taking cancer pain as central to my analysis here, I move past such characterizations of pain as so mired in doubt that it disables relations. To the contrary, the ethnographic work of this book is premised for the most part on socialities that have cohered around cancer pain in Delhi.

To elaborate, in beginning to study socialities of cancer in Delhi, I had to make decisions about which of its constituent practices I would focus on: detection, diagnosis, its various treatment modalities of surgery, chemotherapy, and radiation—these were all possibilities. However, the set of practices I found most striking was the emerging specialization of palliative cancer care and its object of intervention—cancer pain. Palliative care is a biomedical specialization founded on the possibility of understanding, intervening in, and easing pain. In Delhi, where wait times in public hospitals for chemotherapy, surgery, and radiation are often months long, doctors in those hospitals and cancer care NGOs have taken it upon themselves to at least ease the pain that accompanies the disease. By examining this work of palliative cancer care, I describe the many ways pain *is* brought into language, both by those who experience it and those who seek to mitigate it. Explaining the practices that have cohered around pain helps reveal the texture of practices through which cancer is experienced and treated in Delhi.

My focus on cancer pain raises an important conceptual question: Is this a book about cancer or about one of its peripheral symptoms? Is there something missing in an ethnography about cancer that does not focus on the "core" biomedical practices responsive to the disease—screening, chemotherapy, radiotherapy, surgery, and so on? To the contrary, a central concern of this book is to disrupt this distinction between what makes up cancer's center and periphery. Lochlann Jain describes the pink-ribbonization of cancer in the United States and how private corporations have come to dominate its public representations. Their campaigns ask patients to hope and take responsibility for their disease, without questioning the systems that have consistently failed them.[13] Developing Jain's work, Juliet McMullin wonders about the global limits of hope as an imaginary associated with cancer.[14] She hypothesizes that in places where treatments are even more inaccessible than they are in the global north, a concern for pain rather than an embrace of hope might make up the disease's dominant trope.[15] In centering pain, I explore precisely an imaginary and experience of cancer that depart from those associated with cancer in the global north. I center pain because in parts of the world where treatments remain inaccessible, the condition is often an inescapable companion to the disease. Thus, much in the same way that oncologists stress that the category "cancer" suggests a false uniformity when in fact it is a collection of disorders, I argue that taking apart what cancer means unravels the boundaries between the "core" of the disease and its "peripheral" symptoms.[16]

Writing about dialysis in Belize, Amy Moran-Thomas describes how while in many parts of the world the practice is considered a holding measure until transplant treatment, in Belize, a country where no renal transplant has yet been performed, dialysis was reconfigured as a holding measure against death. She describes her ethnographic work, then, as an effort to "remain with these long-term maintenance projects."[17] Similarly, for many patients I spoke to, cancer pain was not a side effect to be treated while curative treatments were enacted. Because of structural difficulties in accessing therapies, pain treatments were often the only form of cancer care they would receive. My effort here to examine pain thus resembles Moran-Thomas's focus on the durability of chronic conditions when treatments remain inaccessible, demanding efforts to endure without the promise of recovery.

Such an approach, focusing on the collections of meaning that have cohered around cancer in one part of the global south, pushes us to rethink its tropes in the global north. That is, even as some public health experts foreground an "epidemic" of cancer pain in lower- and middle-income countries, others point to a simultaneous undertreatment of cancer pain in the United States and Europe.[18] I argue that the underanalysis of cancer pain in places in the global north is a consequence of the overwhelming discourse of hope and survival that envelops the disease. Thus, I show how centering cancer pain forces an acknowledgment of messy realities otherwise obscured by campaigns that "pink-wash" the many inequalities that contribute to its etiologies, prevalence, and consequences. In this way, centering pain in an analysis of cancer is demonstrative of what Jean and John Comaroff call "theory from the south."[19] Thinking through cancer pain offers an opportunity to clarify the *collective* stakes of this condition not only in Delhi but also in other parts of the world where, as Jain and others have shown, its realities have been obscured by tendencies to proselytize its eclipse through individual willpower.[20]

In the same way I do not claim cancer pain is a problem only for the global south, I also do not claim that imaginaries of hope and survivorship are absent in India. The boundaries between the global north and south are hardly ever so clear. The NGO I worked with, Cansupport, organized "Walk for Life" events in the city that resembled similar gatherings of support for survivors elsewhere in the world. However, I found that even such events, oriented toward survival, always highlighted the centrality of cancer pain. For example, in advertising the walks, Cansupport was always careful to emphasize that its primary mandate was "adding life to days, *not* days to life." That is, rather than offer patients the false hope of survivorship, Cansupport workers aimed to make patients' last days meaningful and painfree. If most cancer patients in Delhi present for treatment past the stage of therapeutic intervention, NGOs orient their work toward helping patients live out their last days without pain. During the time of my fieldwork in 2011, Cansupport's founder, Harmala Gupta, described this orientation as a realist response to the context of cancer care in India: "Is there any point in investing our limited resources in more and more expensive and futile treatments when the majority of our cancer population is unlikely to benefit from them?"[21] Citing studies by the *Lancet* and the *Economist*, she critiqued the blinkered search for an elusive cure as "a path strewn with broken promises, dashed hopes, crushed lives and public health systems that can no longer cope."[22]

Echoing Gupta, a palliative care professor at another leading regional cancer care center in South India described his mission against cancer as a second "freedom struggle." If the first freedom struggle secured India's independence from colonial rule, this second would win freedom from cancer pain.[23] The nationalist metaphor of a freedom struggle reveals a pervasive belief among palliative care specialists that India lags behind the rest of the world in cancer pain treatment. They are not alone in this belief; public health experts echo this concern about an untreated pain epidemic in lower- and middle-income countries. A report commissioned by the *Lancet* and authored by some of the most prominent names in global public health begins with the testimony of an Indian palliative cancer care physician and is followed by this editorial comment: "Poor people in all parts of the world live and die with little or no palliative cancer care or pain relief. Staring into this access abyss, one sees the depth of extreme suffering in the cruel face of poverty and inequity."[24] The same study found that in 2015 alone, about twenty million people in lower- and middle-income countries died with serious pain and most of them without access to pain relief. A similar report commissioned by the American Cancer Society in 2013 put the number of global HIV and cancer deaths with end-of-life pain at 2.3 million.[25] Such reports find India at the center of the global pain epidemic. For example, the American Cancer Society report claimed that about 24 percent of these deaths happened in India alone, singling the country out as having the highest incidence of untreated cancer pain. Likewise, journalistic accounts that report on the global pain epidemic focus on cancer in India. Reports in the *New Yorker* and by the BBC restate a statistic that is ubiquitous in such writings: that while India produces most of the world's licit opium, restrictive drug laws deny opioid analgesia to all but about 2 to 4 percent of its cancer patients.[26]

I share this public concern for the undertreatment of cancer pain in India. Much of my work in this book focuses on the experience and treatment of the condition. But I also argue that much like the preoccupation with hope and survival in the United States, there is nothing obvious about the centrality of pain in the biomedical imaginary about cancer in the region. Instead, along with other historians and anthropologists of pain, I show how examining the condition reveals broader assumptions about human vulnerability and social hierarchy.[27] For example, while studying the research literature produced by the growing number of palliative cancer care specialists in the country, I found them preoccupied with the heightened capability of the Indian body to withstand pain. This literature presumed that spirituality and religion were particularly salient in Indian cultural life and hypothesized that they could be instrumentalized as coping mechanisms. Further, experts concurred that any biomedical research on pain among cancer patients needed to account for the role of Indian spirituality. To understand this research orientation, I trace its resonance and roots in several directions. These include the interest of doctors at AIIMS in the new age Art of Living movement and a history of research as old as the institute on spiritual practices to transcend pain. In examining this orientation, I was struck by how much this research resonated with British colonial ideas about Indian bodily dispositions. Historians of colonial India describe the obsession of European writers and colonial officials with the ability of mystics, ascetics, and the *sati* (widows who immolated themselves on their husband's funeral pyre) to withstand pain.[28] These colonial accounts constructed the Indian native as radically different, oriented to a religious transcendence of this world. I do not suggest that there is an unbroken line of continuity from the eighteenth century to the present in social understandings of pain. But I compare these historical and contemporary discourses about pain to explore how cancer research risks depoliticizing the disease. That is, I ask whether this pervasive desire to find ascetic pathways to transcend pain obscures the socioeconomic distributions of the condition in Delhi.

However, despite the limitations of this research paradigm, I found that *in practice*, palliative cancer care practitioners inquired with sophistication into the biological, psychological, and familial etiologies of pain. The multi-modality of pain—its varied etiologies and treatment possibilities—offered pain practitioners a productive site for blurring the line between symptom and disease, the critical and the chronic, and the biological and extra-biological etiologies of suffering. In outpatient clinics, home-care visits, and hospitalized care, pain physicians demonstrated expert knowledge of how neighborhood and kin relations exacerbated or eased cancer's distress. Take, for example, a condition I describe later in the book—phantom limb pain (pain in amputated limbs). The experience of phantom limb pain has been a critical concern in global biomedical pain research. Its intractability has mystified pain physicians for more than a century. One ascendant biomedical pain theory, the neuromatrix model, stakes its validity on its claim to offering the first solution to the problem. Its proponents argue that pain exists as an image in the brain as a neuronal matrix, thus living on in the body even after the amputation of its prior site in the physical limb. Based on this theory, the model offers the device of the mirror box as a treatment. The mirror box reflects a present limb where the absent one should be, tricking the brain into exercising and releasing the pain through this virtual proxy. Yet, as seductive as the neuromatrix theory is in abstraction, ethnographically following a cancer patient with phantom limb pain led me in a quite different direction. This patient's pain biography was more than a decade long. Pain specialists across the city were well acquainted with the intractability of his pain and the failure of a range of treatments. Physicians I worked with had tried the mirror box and many other anesthetic interventions. The thing that had provided the patient in question with the most relief, however, had been high doses of morphine. But rather than dismiss his pain as a lie masking the cravings of an addict, the more experienced specialists maintained their relationship with him, treating him while acknowledging the limits of what they could do. In stark contrast to the imagination of the mirror box that promised a miraculous cure by relocating pain in the brain, these pain physicians understood pain as part of a social relation between themselves and their patient.

Across several sites, then, I came to see that to communicate cancer pain required staking a capacity for belief, even in the presence of suspicions and doubt. It was no surprise, therefore, that pain physicians at AIIMS took a keen interest in its "psychosocial" dimensions, hoping to track down its extrabiological etiologies. At the same time, these expert interventions into the social etiologies of cancer pain hardly solved the problem of pain's unequal distribution. Empathy, in all its forms, could not address the problem that the pain many patients experienced could have been mitigated with timely access to treatment. Further, the small number of trained pain specialists and workers meant that only a small fraction of those needing analgesia received it. Thus, in their capacity for empathy, cancer pain physicians showed both the possibilities and limits of medicine at its most humane.[29] Even as they expressed their capacity for empathy for many individual patients, they could do little to fix the collective inequalities that produced more pain in some rather than others, or the structural limits that put analgesia beyond the grasp of most.

A Disease of Civilization

In discussions about the rise of cancer in India, journalists and scholars often conflate the uncontrolled growth of cancer cells with the recent, rapid growth of the Indian economy. Articles in scientific journals such as *Nature* have claimed that cancer is "a disease of growth" linked to increased affluence.[30] Similarly, newspapers have found that "most cancers in India are caused by lifestyles gone awry" and an outcome of the country putting "economic growth above all else."[31] Medical journals also link a new exposure to international markets with an increased exposure to cancer, while reports from the World Health Organization (WHO) find that cancer is now no longer a "Western" disease but has for the first time entered the developing world on an epidemic scale.[32] The agenda-setting American Cancer Society urges policy makers to look beyond aging and population growth for an explanation of the exploding cancer epidemic in low- and middle-income countries. Specifically, it asks for research on "behaviors and lifestyles associated with economic development and urbanization."[33] Here, I examine this trope of cancer as a new epidemic in India, brought on by lifestyles and behaviors after rapid socioeconomic change. I discuss this trope to demonstrate how it misrepresents the history of cancer in the region and obscures the disease's stakes in the present.

The most recent iteration of the narrative of cancer as a Western epidemic spreading to the non-Western world took shape around the end of the twentieth century, when several global health organizations and experts announced a collective mea culpa. Specifically, they regretted that their long-standing focus on infectious diseases had blinded them to the rise of non-communicable diseases (NCDs) as global health problems. A few scholars took a long view, understanding that NCDs and infectious diseases had always been a simultaneous problem, and that the recurrent panics around infectious epidemics had created a myopia about diseases like cancer.[34] In other words, these scholars recognized the mistake of creating an artificial divide between diseases of the rich (NCDs such as cancer and heart disease) and diseases of the poor (infectious diseases such as HIV-AIDS, tuberculosis, and malaria).[35] However, most public health experts and organizations did not adopt this more measured response; instead, they described NCDs as another *new* precipitous epidemic, much like the ones that had come before. Rather than take the lesson that seeing through frames of crises had narrowed their vision, they replaced an old catastrophe narrative with a new one.

David Jones and Jeremy Greene place this contemporary panic about NCDs within a long history of what they call "public health catastrophism."[36] They describe how such catastrophic narratives project messy contemporary data into the past and future, shaping health policies around pronouncements of ever-repeating crises. Similarly, Carlo Caduff's ethnography of the influenza pandemic shows how such pronouncements concentrate prestige and authority in the hands of experts.[37] The contemporary panic about cancer takes its place within this long history of catastrophic pronouncements of health crises. To locate the starting point of this particular catastrophe, experts mark 2010 as a turning point—the year cancer is said to have outstripped heart disease as the leading cause of death worldwide.[38] Echoing the discourse around NCDs more broadly, cancer catastrophists project a global asymmetry in disease burden; that is, they find mortality rates for cancer rising in lower- and middle-income countries, while rates are in decline in high-income countries.[39] They also find that most cancer cases and deaths have begun to occur in the less-developed world, with Asia accounting for half of the world's new cancer cases and deaths.[40] As Julie Livingston writes in the context of Botswana, these patterns of global visibility and invisibility about cancer frame possibilities of treatment and exposure.[41] Several organizations have emerged in the wake of this alarm, with most large cancer institutions working in the United States and Europe expanding their operations to include lower- and middle-income countries. The global cancer epidemic is now a key target of intervention in the UN Sustainable Development Goals, the World Bank's Disease Control Priorities, and the 2013 WHO Global Non-Communicable Disease Action Plan.

Within India, journalistic and scientific accounts echo this global alarm about a new cancer epidemic in the global south. International epidemiologists estimate that about 1.1 million people in India were diagnosed with cancer in 2018, accounting for about 6.4 percent of the worldwide cases.[42] The Indian government's own disease surveillance data project even more alarming figures. For example, whereas the International Agency for Research on Cancer (IARC) estimates about 1.21 million new cases of cancer in India in 2020, the Indian Council for Medical Research (ICMR) estimates a dramatically higher figure of 1.73 million, which would constitute over 9 percent of worldwide cases.[43] Of course, the same statistics can be made to tell different stories. When adjusted for India's large population, the high numbers of cancer cases in India do not seem as alarming.[44] There is also no consensus on whether the rise in numbers is in or out of step with demographic changes and population growth. That is, researchers disagree on whether there is indeed a dramatic rise in incidence that cannot be explained by considering an aging and growing population. In fact, two persuasive studies demonstrate that if these factors are taken into account, there really has not been a dramatic rise in the rate of cancer in the last decades.[45] Thus, those wary of the narrative of cancer as a "new" epidemic in India contend that cancer incidence has been relatively steady for decades. This is not to say that they do not believe cancer to be a serious public health problem. They more specifically reject claims of a recent surge in the disease's incidence. At the same time, despite this counterevidence, the deceptively self-evident assumption—that the rates of cancer in India have accelerated dramatically in recent years—has become an unshakable trope in journalistic and scholarly accounts.

I draw attention to this trope because it demonstrates a long-standing historical paradox in discussions of cancer. Throughout the twentieth century and into the present, experts have consistently demonstrated cancer's pervasive presence in India.[46] But despite all the evidence to the contrary, writings about the disease continue to associate it with an imagined West and its so-called modern lifestyles. To elaborate, as early as the late nineteenth century, physicians and public health experts demonstrated that cancer was *not* a "Western" disease, and that its lack or presence could not be taken for granted as evidence of a radical difference between the East and West.[47] For example, in 1888, the resident British surgeon-major in Jaipur contested claims in British medical journals that cancer was a disease of the meat-eating West that did not affect predominantly vegetarian Indians.[48] With his experience of the previous eight years in Jaipur, where he had conducted 102 cancer operations, he claimed not only that cancer was highly prevalent among Indians but also that its presentation in advanced stages was a serious and underappreciated problem in the colonies. In 1904, colonial surgeons presented further evidence of the widespread prevalence of cancer in the British colonies, leading the Prince of Wales to declare that "cancer was not a scourge of civilization" as had been previously thought. Rather, he now understood that the disease was prevalent throughout the empire, even where the "civilizing" colonial mission had not yet succeeded.[49] This realization led in 1904 to the addition of the word "Imperial" to the name of the recently founded British Cancer Research Fund (ICRF). For decades after, ICRF researchers continued to reject the framing of cancer as a disease restricted to the colonial metropole. Even as they contended that the disease in India took on particular traits thanks to "barbaric" native customs, they claimed that susceptibility to the disease was not culturally bound.[50] The ICRF's findings were echoed by the British Indian Medical Service, whose epidemiological studies also found that the incidence of cancer in India was similar to that in Western countries.[51] Similarly, Indian epidemiologists too produced research pointing out the relative equality of cancer incidence across the "East" and "West." For example, two Indian doctors at the King Edward Medical College in Lahore published a persuasive study in 1935 showing that the incidence of cancer in India was about the same as elsewhere in the world.[52] At the same time, despite such studies, many contemporaneous researchers obstinately held on to the idea that cancer incidences were and had always been low in India. For example, after surveying the extant epidemiological data, the famous American statistician Frederick Hoffman found that despite the evidence, he could not bring himself to "escape the conviction that cancer in its different forms is unquestionably relatively very rare throughout India."[53]

At the same time, a few voices insisting on the importance of cancer as a health problem in India proved persuasive enough to lead to the foundation of the Tata Memorial Hospital in Bombay in 1940. Founded by the Tatas (one of India's first and most successful capitalist families), the sixty-bed facility was one of the earliest anywhere in the world to combine treatment and research. By 1951, V. R. Khanolkar—president of the International Cancer Research Commission from 1950 to 1954 and a senior oncologist at the hospital—would call it the premier cancer institute in the East. Kavita Sivaramakrishnan describes how Khanolkar pushed against the persisting assumption of the relative unimportance of cancer in India.[54] Instead, establishing a network of support with colleagues worldwide, he argued for a "sameness" in cancer disease rates across the world.[55] India's first health minister, Rajkumari Amrit Kaur, was a prominent supporter of the India Cancer Society.[56] In a 1952 speech inaugurating a session of the International Cancer Research Commission, she claimed that data gathered by Tata Memorial researchers showed that "Indians are as susceptible to cancer as the inhabitants of Western countries and that its incidence is as frequent here as elsewhere."[57] Soon after, she called a press conference to draw attention to the alarming rise in cancer cases in the country.[58] In this "emergency" address, she estimated 200,000 annual deaths to the disease, and its incidence as high as one in every six Indians. In her last two years of her decade-long tenure as the national health minister, she convinced the central government to take control of Tata Memorial Hospital, with the aim of extending its capacity.[59]

The history of cancer in India is thus driven by this curious paradox. On

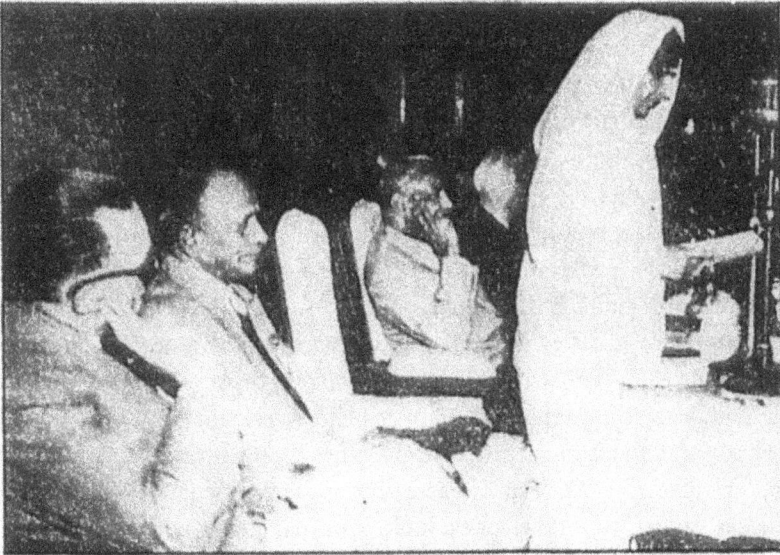

WORLD CANCER EXPERTS MEET

A meeting of the International Cancer Research Commission was inaugurated in Bombay on Tuesday by the Union Health Minister, Rajkumari Amrit Kaur, who also declared open the Indian Cancer Research Institute. Seen in the picture, from left to right, are Prof. J. H. Maisin, Dr. V. R. Khanolkar, Dr. John Matthai and M. Justin Godart. Rajkumari Kaur is addressing the gathering. (*Supplement on pages 8 & 9*)

FIGURE I.1 Health minister Amrit Kaur speaking at a meeting of the International Cancer Research Commission in 1952. Image from the British Library Board Asia, Pacific and Africa sm 77 *Times of India* (Bombay).

the one hand, studies and reports throughout the postcolonial period continued to raise alarms about the disease's critical explosion in India. In 1969, for example, the *Times of India* claimed without evidence that the disease claimed 425,000 lives annually, an estimate that suggested that cancer was more prevalent at that time in India than it is in the present.[60] Even after decolonization, international health agencies continued to warn the Indian government that the incidence of cancer in the country was steadily on the rise.[61] On the other hand, despite these alarms, the myth of cancer as a disease of the civilized West has been difficult to dislodge.[62] Sivaramakrishnan describes the pervasiveness and persistence of the belief among experts and policy makers in the postcolonial period that cancer was a disease of the "West."[63] She also describes how, much to the disappointment of those like Khanolkar who had advocated for a comprehensive cancer program in India, the postcolonial government was instead drawn to developmentalist goals such as population control.[64] Thus, despite the many studies and pronouncements of a cancer crisis throughout twentieth-century India, the myth of cancer as a disease of the West proved an unshakable trope. As a result, infrastructural efforts to treat the disease have remained piecemeal and provisional, limited to a few hospitals in the country's urban centers.

This persisting trope continues to shape contemporary framings of the disease. If cancer is a disease of the West, the story now goes, then its rising incidence must have something to do with the region's increasing westernization. And if this is indeed the case, the disease must disproportionately concern a newly prosperous, westernizing elite. Take, for example, a leading contemporary public health account of cancer in the developing world. This account takes as self-evident the notion that in India "a new middle class has embraced a 'Western' lifestyle characterized by western habits such as high-fat diets, reduced physical activity, increased alcohol consumption and tobacco smoking. Not surprisingly, there has been a surge in the incidence and prevalence of 'Western' diseases such as cardiovascular disease, hypertension, cancer."[65] Or take, for example, a journalistic account of the disease in 2015 that began with the headline "In an Ominous Sign, India Transits Speedily from Infectious to Lifestyle Diseases."[66] Reports such as these identify post-1980s economic growth as the chief culprit for the supposed acceleration in cancer rates, assuming that new "modern" lifestyles adopted by a recently prosperous middle class are responsible for the rise in incidence. In identifying a "speedy transition" to lifestyle diseases such as cancer, this journalistic account looked to public health theories to substantiate her claim. Specifically, she turned to American epidemiologist Abdel Omran's theory of a global "epidemiological transition."[67] In its simplest terms, this theory maps diseases onto progressive civilizational stages. It argues that each society goes through three ages—the age of pestilence and famine, the age of receding pandemics, and the age of degenerative and man-made diseases.[68] As it appears in this journalistic account, the idea perfectly explains the rising rates of cancer in India; cancer is part of the third civilizational age, and westernization is its "man-made" catalyst. In other words, the article presents what is now almost public health dogma: that recent socioeconomic change is a key causative agent in an explosion in cancer rates in places like India. Such accounts present a picture of cancer as a disease of a prosperous Indian middle class that cannot absorb the shock of new social transformations. Their bodies, unable to assimilate rapid modernization, become particularly susceptible to chronic diseases such as cancer. This article's final sentence succinctly captures the troubling implications of such arguments: in the fight against cancer, "there is a lot that is up to one person—you." That is, if a turn to Western lifestyles among an elite few is at the heart of the cancer epidemic, then it follows that correctible behaviors must be at fault, and that the response to cancer must be one of individuals taking responsibility for their self-harming decisions.

Cancer is not the only disease that is framed in such a way in India. Lawrence Cohen writes about how the supposed abjection of old people in postcolonial India became a sign of the decay of an authentic Indian society and the seductions of a putative Western modernity.[69] Cohen describes how experts and policy makers concerned with aging assumed that the traditional Indian joint family had been in decline since the 1980s, and that with the advent of "Westernization, modernization, industrialization and urbanization," aging had suddenly become an alarming problem threatening the country's future.[70] More recently, Harris Solomon has shown how diabetes is similarly configured in popular Indian and scientific accounts as a disease of economic prosperity and modernity, as obese bodies become signs of a failure to metabolize a fast-changing world.[71] I argue here that much in the same way as aging and diabetes, cancer has become a new subject of discussion and intervention, with journalists and experts taking for granted that "westernized" lifestyles are behind the disease's rise. Much like those other NCDs, cancer appears in journalistic and scientific accounts as a marker of the new and a paradigm of an unassimilable modernity. Framed as such, it generates presumptions about the inability of Indian bodies to adapt to social and relational change.

This book has emerged in response to the consequences of framing cancer through such developmentalist tropes. Specifically, I find that these tropes have two dangerous outcomes. First, framing cancer as a disease of a prosperous urban elite legitimizes the absence of cancer care for India's rural and urban poor, when in fact the disease does not respect regional or class lines. A comprehensive study of the distribution of cancer based on 2014 data showed that even though there was a higher prevalence of cancer in urban India, it was also widespread in rural areas that had little access to treatment.[72] Within urban areas, the disease spanned income groups, affecting the city's rich and poor. Further, cancer not only affected both the rural and the urban, the rich and the poor, but also had the ability to *make* poor.[73] In my fieldwork primarily (but not only) among the urban poor, I found several patients driven to distressed financing, incurring financial debts and selling assets to afford treatments or hospitalization. In its ability to make poor, cancer outstrips every other disease; a recent study found that 79 percent of

Indian cancer patients had been driven to catastrophic health expenditures, a number far higher than for any other disease.[74] Thus, framing cancer as collateral damage for postliberalization economic prosperity obscures the prevalence of the disease among the already economically marginalized as well as those driven to poverty after diagnosis.

The second reason that the trope linking cancer to behaviors and lifestyles is troubling is because it places blame on patients rather than on failed health care systems. Khanolkar's postindependence suspicion that the government would not focus its infrastructural energies on cancer proved well-founded. In 1975, the Indian government inaugurated the National Cancer Control Program (NCCP) to build treatment infrastructures and expand access to care. However, the program was soon plagued by charges of corruption. For example, a significant portion of the funds allocated to the program were diverted; out of a budgetary provision of 142 crores in 1984, only 82 crores were used and accounted for.[75] National grants were diverted to other programs, while state governments delayed the release of the funds that were available. In a testament to low expectations, an erudite piece on the state of cancer treatment in 1980 *celebrated* the fact that there were six major hospitals in the country equipped to provide surgery, radiation, and chemotherapy.[76] Soon after, Darab Jussawala (Khanolkar's colleague and his successor as director of Tata Memorial) pointed out the insufficiency of having just ten cancer treatment centers in the country, criticizing the NCCP for having failed in its mandate to build treatment infrastructure.[77] By 1985, only ten years after its founding, the NCCP announced a shift in priorities away from expanding access and toward awareness programs directed at early detection and prevention. While early detection and prevention are laudable aims, they also achieve the effect of diverting attention away from systemic infrastructural lack and toward individual behaviors. As Lochlann Jain suggests, the fetish of early detection obscures the cost and accessibility of treatment, erasing the underlying politics of the disease.[78] Rather than scrutinizing the failures of public health, the NCCP's move distracts from its long-standing failures in bolstering hospital infrastructures.

Further, pinpointing behaviors and lifestyles as causes and promoting early detection as the answer shift the burden of responding to the disease onto already vulnerable patients. For example, the current National Institute of Cancer Prevention and Research guidelines emphasize how new lifestyle choices such as alcohol consumption, overwork, meat eating, and sexual promiscuity are primary risk factors for cancer. In response, this apex governmental body promotes abstinence from such harmful practices to prevent the disease, in the process urging early detection and screening as secondary measures if the first line of defense fails.[79] For another example, the most comprehensive government report on cancer care in postcolonial India begins with messages from the prime minister and health minister urging behavioral correction as an answer to this new "lifestyle" epidemic brought about the "plagues of modernity." The report rehearses old tropes that cancer is a consequence of "Western" practices of drinking alcohol and eating meat.[80] This report then approvingly cites the government's historical shift away from treatment and toward prevention as the correct response to the disease and its thus-identified etiologies. This thrust of governmental cancer policy appears most succinctly in a 2005 *Lancet* article coauthored by officials at AIIMS, the Indian Council for Medical Research, the WHO, and the contemporaneous national minister of health: "As chronic disease epidemics gather pace in India . . . [h]ealth systems need to be reoriented to accommodate the needs of chronic disease prevention and control, by enhancing the skills of health-care providers and equipping health-care facilities to provide services related to health promotion, risk detection, and risk reduction."[81]

Further, the overwhelming focus on early detection and prevention not only places the burden of responsibility for seeking scarce treatments on already vulnerable patients, but also sets patients up for disappointment. As one prominent cancer researcher put it: "Early detection and awareness initiatives of the NCCP may give rise to a rather piquant situation wherein the demands on cancer departments and hospitals may increase exponentially. . . . If the cancer diagnosis and treatment facilities are unable to keep pace, the unmet demands may lead to disillusionment among patients, physicians as well as health planners."[82] In sum, the focus on cancer as "a disease of civilization" and behaviors distracts from infrastructural lack, at the same time as it places responsibility and blame on already vulnerable patients. In a chapter on cancer memoirs, I describe how the callousness of this discourse enters patient memoirs, as writers internalize accusations flung at them by physicians, family members, and neighbors about their cancers being their own fault. Many write about being accused of bad lifestyles and negligence right from the moment of diagnosis, regardless of the type of their cancer and whether it was detectable or treatable in the first place. Such accusations recur most frequently in the accounts of women patients who were often told that their "modern lifestyles" and the stress of entering the workforce had brought on their disease.

Further, in the ethnographic chapters of this book, my descriptions of cancer in India aim to counteract this trope that attaches the disease to a newly prosperous elite, picturing it as a problem of lifestyle and behavior and a by-product of modernity.[83] Instead, I show the effects of the disease on the urban poor and the lower middle class, focusing particularly on how they found ways to manage the duress it placed upon their lives. I find that the pervasiveness of cancer has little to do with lifestyle and behavioral faults, and everything to do with a health care system that fails to provide adequate treatment and care. Thus, rather than fault patients for their inability to absorb socioeconomic change, I demonstrate their inventive strategies to seek treatments and maintain networks of social support, so that they might endure in circumstances hostile to their survival. I track their efforts to negotiate kin, manage pain, and strategize speech, all the while demonstrating capacities for endurance that directly contradict assumptions about their class, lifestyles, and behavioral inflexibilities. Thus, moving away from a paradigm of representing cancer patients as marked by behavioral failure, I present the many ways my interlocutors strove, with varying degrees of success, to absorb the diagnosis into their everyday lives.

Aesthetic Flights

If in my face-to-face ethnography I found a reticence to speak about cancer, in films and memoirs from the region I found instead a profusion of speech about the disease. These aesthetic accounts took the fragility of social worlds around cancer as their theme, staking their own narrative claims about the effects of the disease on social life. My method in engaging these aesthetic efforts is not exactly ethnographic, in that I do not track people's engagement in producing and receiving them.[84] Instead, I am interested in their narratives as complex texts that themselves externalized, critiqued, and reflected social patterns and processes.[85] In exploring films and memoirs, then, I think of them as active attempts alongside my own to imagine and dramatize the ethical stakes of living with cancer.

At the same time, the efforts of many of these aesthetic accounts differ from my ethnographic work in one important respect. If during my ethnography I found no easy answers to the ethical dilemmas provoked by a cancer diagnosis, films and memoirs were much more forthcoming about the lessons that might be learned from an encounter with the disease. For example, in films about cancer, dying patients left behind lessons for other characters and the audience on how to die with dignity, giving their death meaning. For their part, patients in memoirs proselytized the power of in-

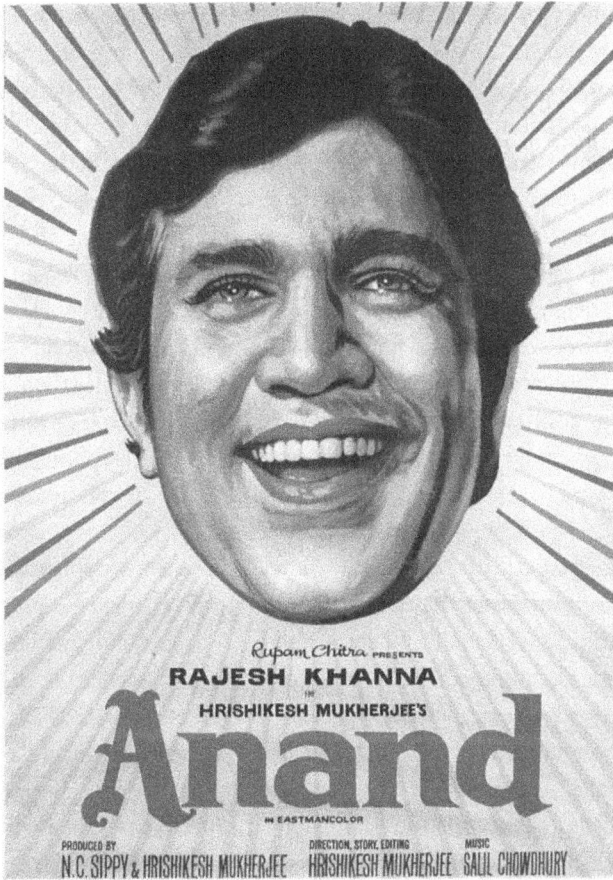

FIGURE I.2 Film poster for *Anand* (1971), arguably cancer's most famous aesthetic account in India. Image from the Osianama Research Centre Archive, Library and Sanctuary, India.

dividual willpower to transcend the disease's suffering, promising survival and joy as rewards for personal resilience. Thus, films and memoirs tended to neatly resolve the fragmentation and crises the disease catalyzed, offering lessons and resolutions that did not come so easily in my ethnographic narratives. Juxtaposing these lessons about resolutions against my ethnographic work helps me to clarify, in relief, the many irresolvable breakdowns in the lives of my interlocutors. In exploring these accounts, then, I ask, what is lost in this aesthetic will to pedagogy and resolution? In answering this question, I sharpen my understanding of the fragmentation erased by such aestheticization.

I share this concern about cancer's aestheticizations with many scholars who study the disease elsewhere in the world. Take, for example, the canonical work of Susan Sontag on the problem of abstracting the messy realities of the disease. As Sontag writes in the opening lines of her own cancer memoir, *Illness as Metaphor* (1978), "Illness is the night-side of life, a more onerous citizenship. Everyone who is born holds dual citizenship, in the kingdom of the well and in the kingdom of the sick."[86] *Illness as Metaphor* remains the disease's most famous literary formulation. In the period since the book's publication, the metaphor of the "kingdom of the sick" has inspired two generations of doctors, patients, and kin to produce memoirs and films about their experience with cancer. However, Sontag herself expressed displeasure that her words had inspired writings about the disease. She wrote later of this opening as "a brief, hectic flourish of metaphor, in mock exorcism of the seductiveness of metaphorical thinking," and of the book itself as an attempt "to calm the imagination, not incite it."[87] She summed up her book's purpose just a few sentences after the opening: illness was *not* a metaphor, and the most truthful way of regarding illness was one purified of metaphoric thinking.[88]

For Sontag, damaging cultural tropes associated with cancer—depressive personalities, military warfare, terrorism—had already hurt cancer patients for too long. Her aim in writing her memoir had been to persuade readers to escape such metaphors and confront the biological consequences of the disease. Ironically, however, despite Sontag's warnings, metaphors and aesthetic productions about cancer have flourished, drawing upon her formulation for inspiration. This flourishing afterlife of Sontag's metaphor, despite her warning against its use, reveals a fundamental tension in representations of disease. Literary scholars criticize the genre for metaphors that abstract away from the suffering caused by the disease.[89] But such critical disapproval has not thwarted the genre's popular success. In the early twentieth century, illness memoirs had a marginal place in literary production.[90] Contemporary memoirs, in contrast, have become one of the most reliably successful commercial genres.[91]

My work draws upon Sontag's impulse to remain wary of cancer's aestheticizations, at the same time as it departs from her normative goal to cleanse representations of illness of all cultural metaphors. Instead, my work here joins other anthropological efforts to delve into such metaphors for what they reveal about the disease's social and cultural life. For example, in her ethnographic memoir, Lochlann Jain examines contemporary representations of cancer in the United States across a range of media.[92] As an anthropologist, she understands her task not as one of "freeing" illness from these cultural metaphors—as Sontag would have it—but of examining them for what they reveal about the worlds in which the disease appears. Similarly, my aim here is to explore the many "cognitive dissonances" (to borrow Jain's phrase) produced by cultural representations of cancer. That is, I describe the vast fissure between the aesthetic abstractions of the disease and the messy experiences of living with cancer. For example, despite the pedagogy of transcendence proffered by many aesthetic representations, the ethnographic stories I tell show how such escapes were only available to very few. In the simplest terms, diagnosis for most of my interlocutors came too late for treatment, giving the lie to aesthetic accounts that proselytized individual willpower and personal strength as the primary preconditions for survival.

At the same time, I also find that a blanket scholarly suspicion toward illness narratives misses the point.[93] Living with the everyday stakes of caring for her ill husband, the literary scholar Ann Jurecic found herself dissatisfied with the all-too-easy critical dismissal of cancer representations. Instead, her experience led her to wonder whether it was possible to define critical practices that were at the same time critical and compassionate.[94] In other words, Jurecic argues that a suspicion toward such narratives risks a disengagement with what aesthetic genres might offer to those who live with critical illness. Here, my way of remaining open to the promise of aesthetic accounts of the disease is to foreground those that hesitate in their search for narrative resolution and restitution. Certainly, some cancer representations I describe here reproduce the same, unsatisfying narratives of personal growth and willed transcendence that have drawn justifiable scholarly ire elsewhere in the world. At the same time, some depart from this trope, describing practices of endurance that rarely resolve in easy recovery and restitution. These accounts offer multiple, fragmented, and even contradictory accounts of everyday life with the disease. In remaining partial and incomplete, they offer a picture of the irresolvable contradictions involved in living and dying with the disease. The main felicity of such accounts is that they do not resolve whether the tragedy they describe is cancer, or the fraught social worlds in which the disease appears. That is, they do not separate out life after diagnosis (the kingdom of the sick) from the life lived before (the kingdom of the well). Rather, they entangle already damaged personal biographies and familial histories with the violence of a new life-threatening diagnosis. Because of this entanglement of past, present, and future vulnerabilities, resolutions in these accounts are never easily at hand. I take these specific genre-resistant films and memoirs as intertextual to my own, offering a set of adjacent entry points with which to understand the lived experience of my interlocutors.

Juliet McMullin examines graphic novels about cancer in the United

States in a similar way.[95] The ubiquity of cancer narratives in popular culture leads her to ask: What can we learn from the narrative work of others about the social relations of cancer? What do these works add to our understandings of stigma, hope, difference, and inequality? Like McMullin and other anthropologists, I find my analysis sharpened in the movement between my own ethnographic text and those aesthetic accounts of disease that stay with the fragmentation in social relations awakened by the disease.

Hesitant Methods

The pervasive reluctance to talk directly and transparently about cancer posed productive challenges to conducting ethnography. These challenges are worth nothing here because they inform the texture and shape of the chapters that follow. In giving me permission to work alongside Cansupport teams, the only condition that the home-care workers put before me was that I be careful about what I said about the disease, to whom, and when. This warning taught me to pay attention to the dexterity with which my informants would both talk and not talk of cancer, describe and deny pain, produce and deny empathy, sometimes all within the same few moments. Guided by the Cansupport teams, I took the methodological tack of witnessing conversations unfold slowly, only rarely intervening with my preformulated questions. While this approach had the limitation of not easily offering systematic answers, it also had the advantage of helping me reframe my attention on subtle practices of care and violence I would have otherwise missed.

To elaborate, in her work on studying performances of mania, Emily Martin draws upon Roman Jakobson's writing about aphasia.[96] Confronted with losing an aspect of linguistic ability, Jakobson saw aphasics as improvising a variety of stylistic maneuvers that were idiosyncratic and yet drew upon the fluidity of language as a social system. In Martin's work, "style" captures both the patterning of social actions and its many indeterminate idiosyncrasies. Styles are personal and particular at the same time as they are social, drawing upon available repertoires of action and behavior. This analytic of style helps me to understand the work of improvisation around cancer as specific to families and patients while at the same time drawing upon the social and political conditions in which the disease emerged. I had to learn through my ethnography to apprehend these many patterned and performative solutions to the problem of language in living with cancer.

Take, for example, the anecdote with which I began this introduction, when our mistake in not hiding the logo "Caring for Cancer" upset a patient. In his naming of his disease as "oncology," this patient was exemplary of many others who preferred to live within a space of ambiguity, rather than inhabit the strict closures that the naming of the disease put into place. Yet, there was no fixed formula on the metaphoric elision of the word "cancer"; such dexterity and concealments took specific forms in every conversation, revealing varied types of context for each negotiation over language. Each ethnographic encounter demanded my pedagogical immersion in this communicative game.

Paying attention to this elision between what was sayable, what could not be said, and what was understood without saying formed the messy site of my ethnographic work. To describe these transactions of words as styles is not to undermine their stakes. The wrong word or gesture could unravel days and weeks of careful work through which my interlocutors sustained their worlds. Mindful of this, if there was one lesson I took away from my interlocutors, it was a lesson in the importance of recognizing my ethnographic limits.

This was never clearer than when I returned to a house where a Cansupport home-care team had visited many times before. This time, they had been called by the family to sit by the bedside of a father who was minutes from passing away. The doctor turned to the family for some holy water from the sacred river Ganga that he pressed to the lips of the patient in his last moments—a gesture toward ritualizing a good death. The son and his wife took part in this shared act. In these last seconds, however, the patient's daughter walked in and, in her grief mistaking the water for morphine, accused the doctor of trying to end her father's life. The team had established a deep rapport with this family, as they had with many others, and they could quickly tap into this reservoir of trust. But while doing so, they quietly sent me away, protecting me as much as protecting the family from the gaze of a relative stranger. The ethnographic lesson I took away from this day was a lesson about witnessing in silence and knowing when to turn away. It is a lesson I hope is reflected in the texture of the work that follows. If I am sometimes reluctant to offer certainty or closure in my analysis, it is because in certain moments, that hesitancy is more faithful to the uncertainties that characterize the experience of critical illness, at a time during which words and gestures sometimes mean more than we know or intend.

Mapping the Book

When I returned home to Delhi in 2011 for fieldwork after spending three years away for graduate school in New York, I noticed signs for several new cancer care NGOs across the city. These included ROKO Cancer, Global Cancer Concern, Indian Cancer Society, CanKids, Cancer Sahyog, Cancer Patient Aid Association, Cancer Aid Society, and the largest and most prominent among them: Cansupport. While some of these NGOs were founded before I had left the city, the number of organizations had multiplied in the years I had been away. Curious about this, I approached the founder-director of Cansupport, exploring the possibility of conducting ethnographic fieldwork alongside the institution's home-care teams. She agreed to my participation, and I was able to follow about ten of the NGO's teams as they provided home-based palliative cancer care to patients. Each team comprised a physician, nurse, and counselor and covered a radius of about fifteen to twenty miles. Over my time with Cansupport, I was able to visit the homes of about a hundred patients who lived across the city. More than half of these patients were among the urban poor who lived in formal and informal settlements. Cansupport staff also introduced me to the director of the palliative cancer care program at the All India Institute of Medical Sciences, which then became the second site of my fieldwork.

The cancer hospital at AIIMS has several teams of specialized cancer experts, an innovative nuclear medicine center, and the latest diagnostic machines and technologies. Its annual budget of about $230 million matched the budgets of many of the best-funded hospitals in the world.[97] With a two-thousand-bed capacity and treating five million patients every year, it is also one of the world's largest hospitals.[98] Writing about ethnographic research at AIIMS thus posed a challenge. As the country's leading hospital, it draws immense budgetary resources from the government and for this reason is hardly representative of many other underresourced public hospitals. At the same time, its reputation attracts patients in numbers beyond its capacity to treat. In this, it resembles many other public hospitals in the country whose infrastructural capacities do not come close to meeting the needs of patients. As will become clear in the following chapter, my description of AIIMS negotiates this combination of its specificity and generality within the Indian biomedical landscape. Rather than taking it as exemplary of Indian health care, I think of this hospital as one entryway into understanding public cancer care in the city.

The chapters that follow are divided by the geography of these sites: the first two come out of my work with Cansupport, and the third is situated at

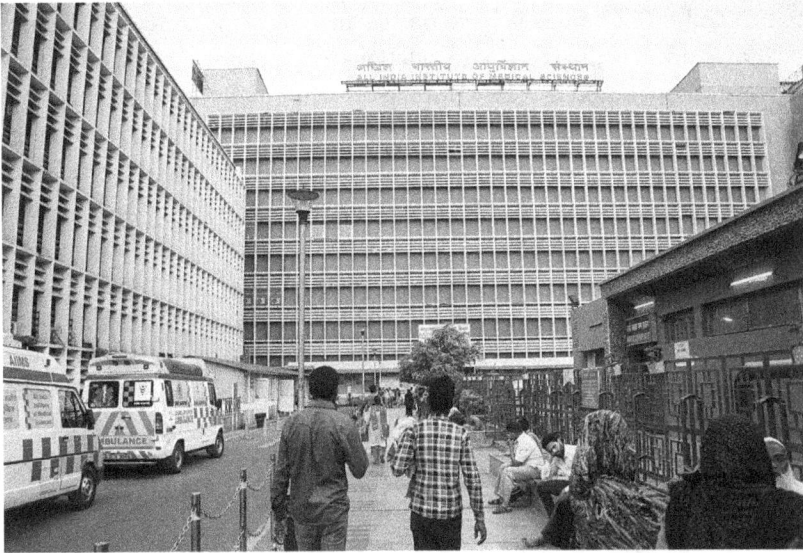

FIGURE 1.3 The All India Institute of Medical Sciences (AIIMS). Photo by Javed Sultan.

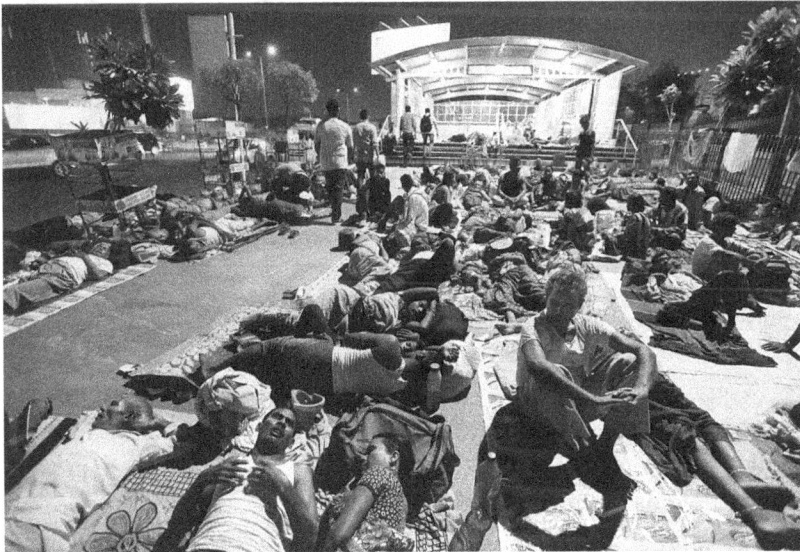

FIGURE 1.4 Relatives of patients sleeping on the pavement outside AIIMS. Photo by Virendra Singh Gosain / *Hindustan Times*.

AIIMS. But they are also divided by thematic and methodological orientations: the first three chapters are based on ethnographic research, while the fourth and fifth chapters depend on the analysis of cultural texts. Consequently, readers with different expectations might choose to focus on different sections of this book. The anthropologically and sociologically inclined might choose to focus on the next three chapters, while those with an interest in the medical humanities might find chapters 4 and 5 closer to their interests. I would urge all readers to end with the concluding chapter, which extends and completes this introduction.

Chapter 1, "Concealing Cancer," focuses on the concealment of cancer diagnoses and its irreducibly multiple textures and implications. For example, concealment for some evidenced care within families. For others, it was a way to safeguard themselves from the harms of revelation, when kin and neighbors hurt rather than aided recovery. I trace the implications of these many motivations and consequences of concealment for palliative care policy, as competing groups of practitioners offered contrasting political models in response to the problems concealment posed for public health work. I also describe an event organized by Cansupport in which family members came together to remember their deceased kin, revealing the importance of concealment in the very moment of overturning its norms. Across these scenes of concealment, I describe it as a strategy to manage the stress that the disease put on social relations. By speaking of cancer only indirectly or not at all, patients and families kept alive a world of an "as-if" in which the disease would not take on the overwhelming force it would gain once named. Through strategic and partial disclosures, they kept alive other ways of relating to family, kin, patients, and neighbors.

Chapter 2, "Cancer Conjugality," tracks the entanglement of palliative care, conjugality, and cancer. I describe how the disease puts pressure on already fraught marital biographies, revealing durable fissures in household relations. As cancer appeared in already broken worlds, it shifted the capacity of husbands and wives to inflict and absorb violence. The debilitating experience of cancer often confined husbands within their homes, making explicit their dependence on the care of their wives. Often, these shifts in the distribution of conjugal vulnerability opened cracks that allowed for long histories of domestic violence and betrayal to seep through. In subtle ways, women could express pasts they had kept hidden and accrue a delicate agency through their practices of care. But at the same time, they continued to inhabit the vulnerable space of affinal homes. I describe, then, how in these conjugal arrangements, empathy, and misrecognition followed each other closely in their tracks, braiding together care and violence to the point of their indistinguishability. I also describe how cancer NGO workers—aiming to treat the social and physical world of their patients—intervened into these broken social relational worlds. In doing so, they found themselves drawn into difficult decisions about how to manage past histories of violence alongside present vulnerabilities.

Chapter 3, "Researching Pain, Practicing Empathy," is based in AIIMS and examines how its doctors produce, treat, and research cancer pain. Physicians at AIIMS who treated pain took an interest in its "psychosocial" dimensions, aiming to track down its social and cultural etiologies. Through these speculative models, they revealed their understanding of how the disease and its social world mutually shaped each other. Their conditional hypotheses about these social worlds demonstrated their efforts at offering a response, however partial, to the constant flow of patients they found themselves responsible for treating. In their responsive capacity for empathy, they expressed a desire to practice a form of humane and humanistic medicine. But even as they showed their capacity for empathy for each individual patient, they could do little to address broader structural inequities that conditioned how pain was socially distributed. Cancer pain, I argue, comes into being in the process of doctors, families, and patients reaching an agreement on how the social and biological etiologies of pain intersect. But I also show how such forms of agreement are hard to reach in conditions of longstanding infrastructural duress that breed doubt about the possibility of pain's amelioration.

Chapters 4 and 5 take cultural representations of cancer in India as their subject. Chapter 4, "Cancer Memoirs," explores how Hindi and English cancer memoirs offer identification and consolation to a new, growing readership in the region. Yet, I describe how such comfort comes at a cost, as many memoirs ask readers to accept responsibility and blame for the disease. These memoirs make the troubling promise of restitution, asking patients to learn to "love their cancer" and relinquish the pessimism that might have contributed to their bodily failure. I describe how I find these generic conventions troubling for laying blame and responsibility on patients rather than on the structural inadequacies in health care that failed them. I then shift focus to memoirs that go against the grain of these generic conventions. Unlike the promise of transcendence offered by accounts of personal responsibility, these explore the durable, and often irresolvable, doubts about social relations that accompany a cancer diagnosis. In doing so, they refuse to draw lines between the precarity of life before and after cancer, showing how the disease folds into already fragile social arrangements.

In chapter 5, "Cancer Films," I describe how, unlike in memoirs, in which cancer patients are urged to live happier lives, patients in Hindi films tend to die. If the dominant affect in memoirs is optimism, cancer films are marked by an overwhelming pathos. Yet, I caution against elite criticisms of cancer films that claim that such portrayals of pathos hinder the happiness of real patients. To the contrary, I find pathos an appropriate mode of representation of a context in which, often, a cancer diagnosis portends death. I find in these films an impulse like my own to investigate the breakdown of social worlds in the wake of a cancer diagnosis. At the same time, if my face-to-face ethnography is concerned with the fragility of everyday life, in these films, cancer becomes a narrative shorthand for a range of imaginations of social crisis—the failure of decolonization, the inability of physicians to live up to their vocational calling, the decline of the modern family, the importance of traditional gender roles, and so on. After identifying these narrative crises, these films tend to resolve them through the death of the patient, leaving other protagonists and the audience with a lesson about the duties of citizenship and personal responsibility. I show, then, how these films—in their will to displacement and resolution—contrast with my ethnographic description, at whose scale ethical resolutions often remained an impossible ideal.

Finally, in the concluding section of the book, "Endurance," I offer some concluding thoughts on the mode of ethics I find characteristic of the practices of my interlocutors. I describe the ethical weight of the effort to carve out a livable life in response to circumstances that do not offer hope. I argue that such a picture of ethical life takes livability rather than flourishing as its potential and horizon. In situations and times that do not readily offer pathways to collectivization and rights, I argue that anthropologists would do well to explore the terrain of everyday ethics committed to enduring in the present. At the same time, in thinking of endurance as ethical, I do not mean that its practices offer a way out of the many impasses of inequality. Instead, I draw attention to the challenging work of maintenance, of folding and absorbing critical illness into everyday life, even in the face of life-threatening duress that continuously invites exhaustion.

1

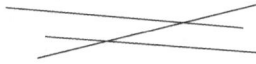

CONCEALING CANCER

Accompanying Dr. Nigam—the head of the palliative care program at the cancer center at the All India Institute of Medical Science (AIIMS)—on one of her ward rounds, I met a twenty-two-year-old man with an advanced malignancy that left him only a few months to live. He had been admitted to the inpatient ward for palliative analgesia. His face revealed little expression, and he remained silent until the end of Dr. Nigam's examination. As she was about to move to the next patient, he quickly called out a question, as if he had been rehearsing it in his mind, "Doctor, why am I in this hospital?" I took it as an expression of existential anger I had heard many times before: Why was *he* in the hospital, why not someone else? Dr. Nigam answered, "Why do you think?" This struck me as insensitive until I heard his response: "There must be some misunderstanding [*galatphemi*]." I had misheard the emphasis of his demand: he had not asked *why* he was in the hospital but, rather, why he was in *this* hospital. In other words, why was he in a cancer ward? He looked away, and after a moment's hesitation and silence, Dr. Nigam turned to the next bed.

Later that day the meaning of this cryptic exchange would become clearer. I was sitting in the doctors' common space when Dr. Nigam gestured me to her office. She had asked the young man's mother and sister to come in to talk with her. After telling them about how he was responding to palliative pain treatment, she asked directly: "How long do you expect him to go on like this? I think he really wants and needs to know; he's asking again and again—why are the doctors not telling me?" His sister's face clouded as she responded: "We don't have the courage [*himmat nahin hain*]." The young patient had been so far shielded from the word "cancer." From the time of his diagnosis a year ago, his family had hidden his disease and its bleak prognosis from him. Dr. Nigam asked in reply: "Do you want me to tell him?" Visibly distraught, the mother responded: "No, he won't be able to take it. We cannot let him lose hope, he will just give up if he knows." Dr. Nigam nodded, but pressed: "I think we should, he will be angry in the future, when the pain gets worse, and he finds out that you knew all along. He is well educated, he will come to understand." Still hesitant, the mother replied: "But don't tell him it's over, that there's no treatment. Tell him we'll still be trying."

In my brief interactions with this family, this was the closest I had found them to speaking the word "cancer." Yet, even without the patient present, they had refused to say the word aloud. I would later find out that for months they had not come to aiims because a sign with the words "Institute Rotary Cancer Hospital" marked the entrance of the cancer ward building. Instead, they had been to two private hospitals where the thicker concentration of departments—often more than one on the same floor—allowed them to avoid ubiquitous signage about the disease. They had, however, been dissatisfied with the pain care at these hospitals and finally came to the palliative ward at aiims. Here, the patient could not have missed the large sign that marked the space as a hospital for cancer treatment when he was wheeled in through the door of the cancer ward building. At the same time, it was unlikely that this was the first time he would have encountered his diagnosis. He was literate, had undergone several rounds of chemotherapy, and had been alone with several other patients with the same disease.

In introducing an important volume on practices of medical disclosure, Mike Davis and Lenore Manderson suggest, "There has been surprisingly little critical attention on how and what people disclose, question and expose, for what purposes, and in what ways."[1] They find this lack surprising, since they understand disclosure as fundamental to clinical practice—always entangled with research, diagnosis, discussions of treatment choices, and prognosis. Their volume is foundational in opening practices of biomedical nondisclosure to anthropological analysis.[2] In this chapter, I develop this anthropological interest in tracking the complex relation between the revelation and concealment of disease, delving into the lived experience of my interlocutors as they inhabited a dynamically unfolding space between disclosure and nondisclosure.

What one told, how, when, and to whom were crucial ways through which the burden of cancer was distributed across social networks, falling more heavily on some than others. In this distribution of speech and silence, awareness of diagnoses and prognoses was never a matter of all or nothing, but a dynamically negotiated site of social transaction. In what follows, I argue that speech and nonspeech about cancer were experiments in social relations. They were strategies through which my interlocutors tested the strength or vulnerability of ties with neighbors and kin, ties whose edges had frayed over time. Importantly, while cancer was often a proximate force that put pressure on these relations, their brittleness also had to do with prior violence that long preceded diagnosis. Here, I show that speech and concealment around cancer are best understood as growing out of these long prior social histories, embedded in the give-and-take of everyday life within which the disease appeared.

To be clear, I do *not* argue that concealment was a way of escaping the significance of the disease or a practice of self-harming denial, as some public health specialists claim. A major limitation of public health debates about medical nondisclosure—including that of cancer—takes its lack or presence as indicative of cultural backwardness or advancement. These framings take nondisclosure as evidence of a culture-bound reluctance in "Asian" countries to measure up to biomedical realities.[3] To the contrary, medical anthropologists Mary-Jo DelVecchio Good and colleagues explain how the norm of disclosure is of recent vintage in the United States, only institutionalized around 1971 with the passage of the National Cancer Act, which shifted the bioethical and cultural consensus from the question of *whether* to tell, to *how* to tell.[4] And, as Cecilia Van Hollen shows, medical bioethicists began to posit telling as normative only after this relatively recent institutionalization of the ideal of cancer disclosure.[5] Van Hollen goes on to argue that with the rise of professional bioethics in the last few decades, the right to autonomy has come to be pitted against "other" cultures where nondisclosure might be contextually appropriate. Rejecting this dichotomy, through her ethnography of cancer among women in Tamil Nadu, Van Hollen describes how her interlocutors were less interested in what information was conveyed or withheld, and more interested in how the act of nondisclosure revealed the care or neglect of those around them. Similarly, in her ethnography of cancer in Botswana, Julie Livingston explains how nondisclosure did not indicate a failure of prognostication, but rather revealed the ethical practice of patients and relatives who took on the burden of discretion as a sign of care.[6] I join this rejection of framing cancer nondisclosure as a sign of cultural lack or medical failure. Rather than take concealment as evidence of biomedical noncompliance, I show that it was a mode through which social relations around cancer were tested, mediated, and reshaped. Specifically, I show that weaving between concealment and speech allowed my interlocutors to inhabit the space of the "as-if," opening the possibility of living in a subjunctive mood. For some, not speaking of cancer opened possibilities of hope. For others, it opened means of persisting in circumstances in which revelation carried danger. I argue, then, that to inhabit this space of the subjunctive was not to escape biomedical realities but, rather, an attempt to make space for the disease *within* already tense social worlds that were newly tested by the pressures of a life-threatening diagnosis.

While secrecy was an ever-present concern at AIIMS, I was able to engage the problem more substantially alongside the staff of Delhi's largest cancer support NGO—Cansupport—with whom I spent time in the homes of about 120 cancer patients. Cansupport was founded in 1996 by Harmala Gupta. She had been successfully treated for Hodgkin's lymphoma as a graduate student in Canada in 1986. The first person to use the "word" cancer to her was a visitor; her doctor had only told her she had "Hodgkin's disease." Gupta remembers not being prepared for the insensitivity with which this visitor named the disease. This incident convinced her of the importance of not "whether you should tell [the diagnosis] but rather *how* you should tell."[7] From that moment on, the importance of the relation between words and illness remained impressed upon her. She returned to India after her treatment and gathered a small group of women to start her work. As the group grew, they began collaborating with AIIMS to offer support to their patients. This informal project concretized into a collaboration with the pain clinic at AIIMS that continues to the present. By the time of my fieldwork in 2011, Cansupport was operating out of thirteen centers in and around Delhi. Its staff included twenty-four teams—each comprising a physician, nurse, and counselor and covering a radius of about fifteen to twenty miles. Within this radius, every team was responsible for about fifty families and patients. About half of these patients had heard of the organization from friends or family and called its help line, while another fourth were referred to Cansupport by doctors at the AIIMS pain clinic. By the organization's own estimates, it had provided care to 746 patients over the year before my fieldwork, with roughly equal numbers of men and women.[8] According to the same estimates, most of these patients were "lower-class" (54 percent), and most others were "middle-class" (38 percent).

Concealment as Care

On one home-care visit with Cansupport, I accompanied a team to the city's eastern border. Rohini—the wife of the patient we were visiting—greeted us on the path leading to her home. She then took us inside, where her husband, Shambu, lay in apparent discomfort in a double bed placed in the center of a small room. Their teenage son was away at school. Shambu had been a door-to-door life insurance salesman who now presented with an advanced stage of prostate cancer. He was the family's sole earner, and two years of treatment had depleted their financial resources. He did still own the plot of land on which his two-room house was constructed. The Cansupport doctor I was with administered to Shambu's pain and enlisted the help of a nurse he knew who lived a few houses away in the neighborhood.

Here, as in most other cases, who knew what was a sensitive matter. We walked outside the house under the pretext of seeing a new provision store in the neighborhood. The counselor's tactful conversation in that time with Rohini elicited that she had an accurate picture of Shambu's diagnosis and prognosis. However, Rohini was certain that while Shambu knew his diagnosis, he was unaware of its prognosis. That is, while he probably knew he had cancer, she believed he did not know how far his malignancy had advanced. She had colluded with the doctor to protect Shambu from the psychic impact of the knowledge of his imminent death. But maintaining this secrecy had been difficult for her, and she was open to the counselor's suggestion that they talk to Shambu about how much he knew and whether he was prepared for the months ahead. Soon we returned to their house, and Rohini left us alone with Shambu. Talking to Shambu revealed that he was not as much in the dark as Rohini imagined. He had spoken to other patients at AIIMS and had learned to read between the lines of clinical conversations. While we spoke to him, no one said the word "cancer" out aloud. We spoke instead of the side effects of his *bimari* (illness) and treatment. Talking with him also revealed that the couple had gravitated toward a new "alternative" cancer hospital in a nearby neighborhood. They had been visiting this hospital over the past few weeks, hoping for a better outcome. The staff there had complied and claimed they could completely cure the disease if Shambu and Rohini paid with all their savings and the proceeds from selling their house. The hospital's promise did not surprise the counselor. She had heard of several such private cancer clinics cropping up around the city, at least some of which crushed steroids and painkillers into small paper pouches and charged high fees. Oncologists at AIIMS knew of these clinics and told me how they often lost patients to the promise of a quick and complete cure. Treatment at AIIMS required long trips across the city and hours, if not days, of queuing on the pathways around the hospital. Encouraged by the rejuvenating effects of the steroid cocktail, many patients would sometimes abandon curative and palliative treatment at the hospital. Cecilia Van Hollen has written of a similar world of "alternative" and "complementary" therapies that emerged in response to the HIV-AIDS crisis at the turn of the century, when promises of complete cures by some alternative practitioners not only discouraged patients from pursuing biomedical treatments but, more dangerously, also led them to believe that they were no longer infectious.[9]

A few days before visiting Shambu, I had spoken with another family facing a similar conundrum. The aging father of that large joint-residence family had been diagnosed with cancer. Hearing of alternative treatments at new cancer clinics, the man's two sons had paused his chemotherapy; the alternative clinic the sons found discouraged them from continuing biomedical treatment. After the short-term benefits of the painkiller and steroidal cocktail had worn off, the effects of the disease returned redoubled. With curative or life-extending treatment no longer an option, the two sons now lived with the regret of having switched treatment modalities. In his work on tuberculosis in India and its history of relapse and drug resistance, Bharat Venkat suggests that sometimes the proclamations of biomedical cures are like promises rather than ruptures.[10] That is, they do not always announce the onset of a healthy future but, like all promises, can come to be broken. In this instance, the promise of a cure not only was broken but also was made in bad faith. The counselor I was visiting with knew of this, but she did not tear down Shambu and Rohini's last hopes for treatment. Later, she told me that directly criticizing such clinics might have risked patients' trust in her; they might read professional jealousy into her effort to discourage them from seeking treatment elsewhere. As the family talked, it became clear that they were considering risking their savings for their son's education to obtain this therapy and selling their small home. Remaining noncommittal on the viability of a cure, the counselor urged Shambu and Rohini to talk through the potential implications of their decision.

Later in this conversation, Shambu and Rohini complained about the treatment they had received at this alternative clinic. The physician there had refused to come into physical contact with Shambu. Instead, their conversation had revolved around the staff determining where the family lived, whether they rented or owned their home, and how much they had saved over the years. The counselor urged them to think about what kind of trust such an interaction could build. Shambu and Rohini first demurred but then revealed their skepticism about the clinic's eagerness to dispense medicine without conducting any tests. The counselor took this opening to tell stories of other patients who had lost their life savings, seduced by the promise of cures. Soon afterward, Shambu again changed the course of the conversation and told the story of his life. As an insurance salesman, he had planned his own life insurance policies based on an astrological prediction that he would contract a life-threatening disease. but that prediction had fallen short by two years and derailed his plans. His guilt at leaving his wife and son without financial means weighed heavily on the rest of our talk.

How might we understand the stakes of the secrecy between Shambu and Rohini? Why did it remain so important to not speak directly of cancer, even as both the diagnosis and the prognosis lay in plain sight? Shambu, Rohini, and the nurse from the NGO all knew Shambu had cancer and that his prognosis was not hopeful. But while they knew, they shared the vital knowledge of knowing what not to say. Knowing what not to say allowed for them to continue to live in the present, without compromising all hope of the future. In their work on illness narratives, Byron Good and Mary-Jo DelVecchio Good call our attention to "subjunctivizing tactics"—stories through which patients, families, and physicians maintain multiple perspectives on disease and possibilities of hope and healing, even when healing would be miraculous.[11] In Shambu and Rohini's life, I suggest, secrecy evidenced a similar desire to live in the subjunctive, to not foreclose possibilities of hope and life even in the face of likely death. Living in the subjunctive allowed Shambu and Rohini to continue their life in the present as if the future was not already preordained. They staked their concealments on their judgment of how much speech the other could absorb and how much they should disclose, when they knew such disclosures could put their relations at risk.

A century ago, Georg Simmel suggested that secrecy was fundamental to intimacy and not its enemy.[12] This was because the possession of full knowledge of the other took away all possibility of fantasy. Thus, according to Simmel, secrecy was implicit in love precisely because love was the possibility of the gift of future revelations. To an extent, Simmel's insight holds true here, as Shambu and Rohini sustained their world through partial concealments and slowly unfolding partial disclosures. Yet, contra Simmel, the function of concealment between Shambu and Rohini was not to safeguard parts of the self for the certainty of a future. Rather, they directed their strategies at the present within which they kept alive the possibility of recovery. They lived in the subjunctive not in the sense that they lived in a false, fantasy world, denying the truth of their biomedical quandary. Returning to the description by Good and colleagues, living with illness often "embodies contradictions and multiplicity," and so its narrative "cannot be represented all at once or from a vantage. It is constituted, rather, as a 'network of perspectives.'"[13] For Shambu and Rohini, secrecy was precisely such a subjunctivizing strategy, a grappling with the incoherence and disruption of cancer by maintaining multiple and even somewhat contradictory points of view, simultaneously knowing and keeping at bay their knowledge of what their futures held. To be clear, this space of hope was not the space of denial or an imaginative transcendence of the messy facts of the disease. The "as-if" was always bound tightly to the real. Both knew the bleak prognosis, both experimented with other possible therapeutic options, but at the same time, both understood the limits of such possibilities. The "as-if" of the subjunctive mood as it unfolded here was not an escapist fantasy but a mode of coping with the ever-present stakes of a threatened real.

The Dangers of Revelation

In Shambu's case, the network of social relations around him afforded support within which Cansupport could work. Despite his difficult financial circumstances, Rohini was a constant presence, they could rely on their son to run errands, and the nurse in their neighborhood would be a consistent resource. For many other patients, however, neighbors and kin often exacerbated their vulnerabilities. In one of my first home visits with Cansupport, I met Rajesh, a twenty-nine-year-old man who had been battling chronic myelogenous leukemia since his teenage years. Rajesh rented a small makeshift room on the roof of the house of his paternal relatives. To reach his room, we had to walk up a narrow, snaking staircase that took us through the lower floors. His family's greetings to us were perfunctory; they were not keen on Rajesh having visitors. Arriving at Rajesh's room, I saw how its walls were bare but for two pictures—one of a Hindu deity (Vishnu) and another of his parents, who had died in a road accident when he was a teenager. Rajesh had contracted cancer soon after his parents' death, while he was working at a chemical factory on the outskirts of the city. The little money they had left him and the wages he had saved were spent in the early months of his treatment. His paternal kin had taken him in but refused to extend any care. In the early days after his diagnosis, his family's resentments saw to Rajesh's isolation in a small, barely covered veranda of the house. Yet, his will to live was strong: he would undertake a difficult journey to AIIMS in the early morning and make himself available for consultations and treatment. Hospital policies at AIIMS dictated that, given the debilitating effects of cancer therapies, patients must always be accompanied by a family member or attendant. To circumvent this requirement, Rajesh would sign his patient forms twice—once under his own name and once again, after leaving the ward and returning in disguise to sign as his own attendee.

Rajesh's family had hidden his diagnosis from their extended kin and neighbors, ensuring their own protection from accusations of neglect. Even if it was not their intent, this arrangement benefited Rajesh. He believed if their neighbors found out about his disease, they would ostracize him, which not only would result in further social isolation but also would exacerbate his financial duress. At the time, Rajesh was earning the supplementary money he needed for his treatment by running errands for many families in his neighborhood. Rajesh was convinced that if they found out about his cancer diagnosis, they would shun him, and he would lose the only income he had. I asked whether it might help if his neighbors found out that his family was neglecting to care for him; would that perhaps shame his kin into extending him some support? Rajesh was not sure that this would be the outcome of his diagnosis becoming public; he suspected that his neighbors might side with the family rather than with him, sympathizing with the family's misfortune in having to take care of an unwelcome invalid.

One way to understand and examine Rajesh's insistence on concealment would be to look for its cause, asking about the cultural beliefs that lead to its practice. Indeed, public health writings about cancer nondisclosures in India focus on the stigma associated with the disease, offering up a typology of cultural misunderstandings about the disease that are believed to contribute to this stigma. For example, many physicians and health experts identify beliefs about cancer—that it is contagious, a punishment for a past sin, or a death sentence—as explanations for why patients are stigmatized and feel the need to conceal their diagnosis.[14] Yet, while such beliefs might well contribute to stigma, this explanation leaves out an important aspect of concealments that primarily interests me here: the prior social worlds within which concealments and disclosures unfold. That is, while practices of concealment might certainly have something to do with cultural beliefs about the disease's etiologies, its consequences and distribution take shape in relation to present social vulnerabilities. Put differently, even as public health scholarship is preoccupied with correcting false beliefs about contagion and moral disorder, neither Rajesh nor his family ever offered such causal explanations for their desire to conceal. When I asked him once why he thought cancer evinced such strong and negative reactions, Rajesh shrugged inconclusively. But when we talked about another cancer patient in the same neighborhood who also kept the disease secret, Rajesh remarked that he did not think disclosure would have the same devastating effect for that person that it would for him. The other person he talked about was the head of his household, had a secure source of income, and had access to officials who could help him obtain state financial aid. The consequences of a forced or unintentional disclosure to the wrong person or at the wrong time would be quite different for the two patients. For the other patient, Rajesh suggested, this might mean only unwanted concern. For himself, it would mean the loss of livelihood, or an isolation even more limiting than what he already experienced. Drawing from my experience in talking to Rajesh and others like him who felt it necessary to keep the disease secret, I suggest that the least understood and most important dimensions of disease nondisclosure are not the cultural stigmas associated with the disease but the shifting, local relational worlds within which the disease appears. In other words, the *why* of cancer stigma (for example, a typology of cultural beliefs) does not help reckon with *how* nondisclosures gather force within a person's world and illness experience. How the disease folds into local worlds depends on the singularity of biographies and the social relations through which a person comes to matter.[15] For Rajesh, his isolation and abandonment had begun long before his diagnosis. If the fear of contagion or an attribution of the disease to his moral failing mattered at all, it was only in how they joined with his already vulnerable place in his world. Cultural understandings of the disease only sharpened the consequences of these long-existing vulnerabilities, whose roots ran deeper than the fact of his illness. Put differently, whereas public health scholars understand the "context" of nondisclosure in terms of stigma and cultural beliefs, I frame it as the interlocking local social hierarchies within which patients are placed.[16]

Remaining attentive to these relational stakes of nondisclosure—when and to whom practices of speech and concealment are dynamically directed—helps focus our understanding of its consequences. As the costs of his treatment escalated, Rajesh's long history of familial isolation and financial vulnerability became increasingly significant. For many patients in the world with financial resources or comprehensive cancer insurance, the first-line treatment for chronic myelogenous leukemia is a pill taken once a day: Gleevec. At the time, the drug was the focus of a legal battle between Novartis—the pharmaceutical corporation behind Gleevec—and the Indian government and was not easily available in Delhi's public hospitals.[17] And, in any case, as Stefan Ecks has explained, the philanthropic patient-access programs developed by Novartis do more to foster a fiction of corporate responsibility than to really expand possibilities of care.[18] At AIIMS, unable to prescribe Gleevec, Rajesh's doctor recommended a bone marrow transplant (BMT). When Gleevec is available, transplants—which often carry a risk of fatality and are associated with far worse outcomes—are now only a last option. Without Gleevec, Rajesh's only choice was to risk the infections, organ damage, and graft failure associated with BMTs. But even accessing a BMT was no simple matter. Because AIIMS is a public hospital, treatments there cost a fraction of what they would in private hospitals. For example, subsidized surgical tumor excisions range from around 3,000 to 13,000 rupees ($50–$200). To offset this cost, showing that one's family income falls under the poverty line makes one eligible for a further fee remission of up to 6,000 rupees ($100). However, the BMT that Rajesh needed fell within a range of interventions (along with others such as cardiac defibrillation, carotid stenting, and hip replacements) that incur prohibitive costs even at AIIMS. While the cost of a BMT in a private clinic can exceed a million rupees ($15,000), AIIMS offered this treatment to Rajesh for about 260,000 rupees ($4,000), a third of the private care price.

For such expensive cancer treatments, the main sources of financial respite are a few government grants redeemable only at the twenty-seven Indian hospitals accredited by the National Cancer Control Program. AIIMS is the hospital in this network that is responsible for covering much of the national capital region. With Cansupport's help, Rajesh had sought these government cancer funds but he was eligible to apply for only three of these grants. The first was administered by the Prime Minister's National Relief Fund, set up in 1948 to aid in the aftermath of the partition of India. Since then, its mandate has grown to include assisting those struck by natural disasters and suffering from noncommunicable diseases. This grant is funded by public contributions and gets no budgetary support. Even though it has the least complicated application procedure, its disbursements are too small to cover the cost of more expensive cancer treatments. The second and third grants—from the State Illness Assistance Fund and the Health Minister's Cancer Fund under the Rashtriya Arogya Nidhi (National Health Fund)—were administered by the Ministry of Health and Family Welfare and given directly to AIIMS. The first allocates about 50 million rupees for "life-threatening" illness, with a maximum of 150,000 rupees per patient. The second—designated for cancer patients—allocates about 5 million rupees to each of the twenty-seven national centers, with a maximum of 100,000 rupees per patient. These discretionary funds allowed AIIMS to subsidize patient costs. But, like many others, Rajesh's treatment exceeded the per-patient allocation. To circumvent this, he would have to apply to the Ministry of Health and Welfare for an individual dispensation. To do this, he had to work with both his treating physician and the head of the department at AIIMS to prove that his disease was immediately life-threatening. This would require several visits to the hospital, all while his disease progressed. Then, he had to demonstrate an income below the poverty line for his entire family, proof of which would need to be attested to by two local political authorities responsible for his neighborhood. For those who lived outside Delhi and had traveled for treatment, this itself was an almost insurmountable obstacle. Rajesh's problem was different. If the income of the extended family he lived with was added on to his own earnings from running errands, he would no longer qualify for government assistance. But since no financial assistance was forthcoming from his family, he would have to approach the district officer and convince him of his situation. To do this, he drew up a document that proved he paid a small rent to his family members. With no income of his own to show, Rajesh visited district offices, seeking assistance from a broker who helped him negotiate the tricky process. At this stage, district clerks and officials could easily hold up his application. This provided opportunities to demand bribes, and Rajesh had to convince them he had no money at hand to give. It took several months before he could submit his application to the Ministry of Health, holding up his treatment because the assistance programs stipulate that they do not reimburse costs incurred before the final receipt of the application. Fortunately, after all this, Rajesh's transplant surgery and adjuvant therapies proved successful.

That Rajesh could negotiate these transactions and prove his eligibility was almost miraculous. During our conversations, he spoke knowledgeably about the intricacies of every bureaucratic procedure he had encountered and the ways he had devised to circumvent the process. Much of this story was of strategic disclosures, of knowing what to say to whom to remain on track for his treatment. In negotiating this process, Rajesh had been aided by the type of his cancer, one that did not require debilitating surgical amputations. He had also relied on the advantage of his youth and his ability to learn the intricacies of the bureaucratic process. Signing under two different guises to access treatment was only one of the many skills that Rajesh had mastered. He also spoke about which doctor at AIIMS was the most pliant and empathetic, about which clerk at the Ministry of Health had been the least corrupt or most likely to help, and about which forms were most vital and which forms could be filled out with less attention to procedural detail. Through his negotiations of this array of governmental processes, Rajesh himself has become a source of expertise. The team I was visiting with deferred to Rajesh's experiential knowledge as they asked for his help in guiding another recently diagnosed young cancer patient. Thus, Rajesh's appearance in the legal and bureaucratic process as an eligible recipient of aid was a hard-earned status. Unsurprisingly, few others could construct their own vulnerability with the proficiency and speed that the disease demanded. At the same time, the long course of Rajesh's illness had exhausted him. Recently, Cansupport had been urging its philanthropic funders to buy a food-vending cart for him, to help secure the monetary independence he needed. Meanwhile, he continued to run errands for his family and neighbors, learning to swallow his resentment and strategically disclosing his diagnosis to some and not to others. At the end of our last conversation, his usually upbeat demeanor collapsed, and he stated bluntly that if the disease returned, he would not fight it again.

Living in the Subjunctive

In Rajesh's world, cancer was a different kind of secret than for Shambu and Rohini. It did not evidence care as much as it constituted a premise of his survival. Such an understanding of the stakes of concealment is important because it pushes against how concealment is often understood by bioethicists, biomedical practitioners, and public health experts: as a sign of medical noncompliance and evidence of escapism. For example, in bioethics discourse, any prevarication about telling diagnoses is understood as a contravention of its most sacrosanct norm—the autonomy of the patient and his or her right to know. As Alex Broom and Assa Doron show, many cancer physicians in India too understand nondisclosure as indicative of ignorance and denial, even as they participate and collude in the act.[19] Yet, I found nondisclosures to evidence neither ignorance nor denial, but rather a way through which patients reconciled the vulnerabilities of their life before and after the disease. Concealing his disease from some and disclosing to others helped patients like Rajesh distinguish between kin, institutions, and physicians they could trust and those that could inflict further harm. At the same time as he sought institutional attention, Rajesh pushed away from the risky gaze of neighbors and kin. At the same time as he made himself visible in the more distal context of AIIMS, he sought invisibility in his proximal world. Rajesh's strategic doubling—of appearing as himself and as his own attendant—was a powerful analytic for the ethical world he inhabited, a world that demanded multiple and simultaneous experiments of staking concealment and disclosure to maintain his place within his proximal social world. As Veena Das puts it in writing about illness in Delhi, the relation between concealment and medical care is thus more complicated than a simple equation of nondisclosure with noncompliance; concealments do not indicate the absence of a desire to find and seek treatments.[20] Biomedical discourses that vilify concealment as an inability to face up to the reality of the disease miss how it was precisely by navigating between concealments and disclosures that my interlocutors found ways to measure the disease's consequences.

Resonantly, in her work on birth and death in rural India, Sarah Pinto writes that biomedical doctors and NGO workers committed to full disclosures misrecognized practices of concealment as a sign of women's ignorance or disinterest in better health.[21] Pinto's ethnography shows instead how acts of disclosure and concealment became crucial to the bodily and moral praxes of her interlocutors, situated as they were within complex social relations of caste and gender. Crucially, Pinto suggests that such acts of concealment were part of a complex push and pull away from and toward authority, a simultaneous evasion of and longing for institutional attention. My approach toward concealment here mirrors Pinto's in resisting explanations that assume Indian patients are somehow incapable of fully grasping the significance of their disease, or that acts of concealment necessarily evidence the absence of health-seeking behavior. Such acts are not "ignorant" of reality, nor do they "normalize" or "deny" difficult circumstances.[22] Instead, nondisclosures reveal how encounters with life-threatening illness are never far away from the experience of everyday life.

The two cases I described here do not exhaust the many forms and functions of concealments in the lives of cancer patients I encountered during my fieldwork. But in each instance, managing illness knowledge played a significant role in shaping the possibilities and trajectories of treatment and care. For Shambu and Rohini, secrecy helped sustain the possibility of living in the subjunctive—in the mode of the "as-if"—performing the hope of survival even with the knowledge of likely death. For Rajesh, too, inhabiting the possibilities of the concealment was a crucial coping strategy: his ability to move between different narrative positions, between disclosure and nondisclosure, aided his survival. Thus, even if practices of concealment varied in motivation, purpose, and consequence, they were always a way for my interlocutors to negotiate proximate others and the textures of support or harm they promised. Concealing helped many to weave the disease into broader concerns of their lives, allowing them to live within social relations in which they found varying degrees of abandonment and support. It became one more way, among others, through which patients, families, and caregivers tested the durability of already frayed social relations put under further pressure by cancer.

It is worth noting here that cancer is not the only disease whose knowledge requires circumspect experiments with speech and disclosure. For example, anthropologists and other scholars of public health have documented the concealment of HIV-AIDS in many parts of the world. For example, drawing from his work with an HIV-AIDS nonprofit organization in Indonesia, Tom Boellstorff describes the disease's association with non-normative sexuality as contributing to a reluctance to name it.[23] Similarly, Kate Wood and Helen Lambert present the disease's nondisclosure in South Africa as a response to its stigma, suggesting that concealment evidenced a desire to avoid the disease's association with sexual promiscuity.[24] My work here joins such writings about nondisclosure as a coping strategy but also departs from them in one important respect. That is, the focus of the literature on HIV-AIDS emphasizes how negative cultural beliefs stigmatize the sufferers of this disease, sharpening the consequences of its nondisclosure. For example, Wood and Lambert describe how their ethnographic interlocutors diagnosed with HIV-AIDS preferred to say they have cancer, as a ruse to escape this stigma.[25] Here, I argue that bringing cancer (a disease not often associated with nonnormative sexual practice) into discussions of nondisclosure pushes us to look beyond the role of cultural beliefs as determinants of stigma. Speaking with interlocutors such as Rajesh helped me to see that nondisclosure was as much a result of fears that disclosure might exacerbate prior vulnerabilities that preceded the illness as it was about negotiating cultural beliefs associated with cancer. In other words, paying attention to the embeddedness of nondisclosure in everyday life helps reveal how familial dynamics, personal biographies, and situated vulnerabilities shape the distributions of speech about cancer.

At the same time, even as I push against the emphasis on cultural beliefs in the HIV-AIDS literature on nondisclosure, I draw crucial insights from that literature. For instance, Lambert and Wood argue that practices of nondisclosure maintain hope and keep alive imagined possibilities of recovery.[26] Closer to the context of my work here, Mathew George and Helen Lambert show how the concealment of HIV-AIDS diagnoses helped patients and families in South India reassert and maintain a sense of normality in their lives.[27] Similarly, in the fraught and unsteady arrangements of my ethnographic contexts within which cancer appeared, concealment allowed for the possibility of thinking and living in the subjunctive, in the mode of the "as-if"—performing the hope even with the knowledge of a likely death.

Developing the work of Adam Seligman et al., Vaibhav Saria argues that living in the subjunctive in times of social failure allows for a temporary respite from broken worlds of experience, producing ways to manage the fractures of everyday life.[28] But Saria also suggests that this escape is ultimately doomed, as the actual returns to make demands on the "as-if." Drawing from Saria's insight, I argue that even as strategic nondisclosures make space for living in the subjunctive, the space of the "as-if" nonetheless remains anchored to the actuality of the disease and the durability of long-standing prior vulnerabilities. Even as Shambu and Rohini made space for contradictory narratives and partial hopes, they remained caught in the uncertain space between the diagnosis and the disease's outcome. I think of concealment here as a strategy that seeks to multiply possibilities of living with the disease, while at the same time remaining aware of its consequences. Living in the subjunctive made possible brief respite from the real, even as such respite often turned out to be temporary, and the "as-if" never really escaped the grasp of the actual.

Modeling Palliative Care

In 2005, a heated debate broke out on the usually placid pages of India's flagship pain and palliative care research forum, the *Indian Journal of Palliative Care*. This debate distilled two different visions of palliative care for India. In the introduction, two palliative care professionals from the International Observatory on End of Life Care at Lancaster University (UK) laid out the terrain of this debate.[29] Drawing on palliative care implementation in many regions of the world, they presented a spectrum of possibilities for delivering palliative care in India. On one end of the spectrum were high-quality, small-scale interventions administered by specialized professionals. On the other were participatory, community-led efforts that provided care through a network of nonexpert neighborhood caregivers. The authors criticized the former model for ignoring how, in conditions of infrastructural lack, an insistence on specialization restricted palliative care to only a small minority of those that needed it. Instead, they lauded neighborhood care for encouraging communities to take control of their own well-being.

The debate that followed in the journal took the side of one or the other model and mapped it onto two different states in India. On one side of the debate were palliative care practitioners from the state of Kerala in southern India. On the other were practitioners from Delhi. Palliative cancer care in Kerala has taken a community-oriented form, led by a coalition of four organizations under the rubric of the Neighborhood Network of Palliative Care. An essay by two founding members of this collective—Suresh Kumar and Mathews Numpeli—laid out the Kerala model.[30] They argued that pain and palliative care were an integral part of primary health care, not an afterthought to assuage the failures of public health. Further, they argued that "emic volunteers" within neighborhoods were best attuned to the needs of patients. The broader political and pragmatic thrust of their argument hinged on their contention that global political-economic conditions have denied most of the world's poor access to medical care, and that in such conditions, community ownership of health care has led to better health outcomes.

Others, however, questioned the success and translatability of the Kerala model. In the forum it drew the strongest criticism from Harmala Gupta, the founder of Cansupport. In a sharp riposte that showed her acquaintance with social theory, she singled out for attack Neighborhood Network's idealization of "communities" and "participation": "There is a tendency amongst us to mourn the loss of a traditional past with its sense of a closely knit and concerned community. Yet, when we look closely at the requirements of palliative care delivery, can we overlook the specifics of the dying patient's deepest needs? Are the interests of this sick person best served by amorphous interventions extended by well-meaning people, perhaps even neighbors, or by trained professionals comprising doctors, nurses, and counselors?"[31] To answer this question, she drew from her experience of founding Cansupport and its subsequent success in Delhi. Her argument rested on the claim that palliative care must be the responsibility of trained professionals. While Cansupport began as a community of survivor volunteers, their work alongside AIIMS had showed to them the need for professional expertise in delivering palliative care. According to Gupta, "We are constantly asked by a number of our patients to park our vehicle at a safe distance, away from the curious eyes of neighbors. It is a request we abide by, as we are only too aware that not only is it a matter of preserving confidentiality but that in our society cancer carries a stigma that can impact negatively on the patient and on the family. It is the reason why people tend to hide the diagnosis even from those closest to them."[32] As presented in her article, neighbors did not appear as disinterested outsiders or a constituency that could easily be mobilized for support. They were people with whom patients had a shared history and sometimes violent pasts. Gupta made a further argument that depression, anxiety, and other comorbid forms of psychological distress that accompany cancer were not illnesses that volunteers were trained to treat. In concluding, she argued that the multimodality of palliative care distress required an equally multipronged response. As an alternative to the Kerala model, she proposed the Cansupport model—care delivered to homes by teams of professionals that included nurses, counselors, and doctors. For Gupta, anything less than such a specialized commitment disrespected the needs of the dying person.

The final word in this special issue raised the global stakes of the debate. It came from Jan Stjernswärd, a legendary name in global cancer care. After decades of work in Africa, Stjernswärd served as the chief of who's cancer program from 1980 to 1996. Near the end of his tenure at who, Stjernswärd had trained oncologists in Kerala in palliative care work, including those who contributed to this journal issue. The Kerala Neighborhood Network model that Kumar and Numpeli defended had been established as a who-funded demonstration project, in collaboration with Stjernswärd. In a biting critique of the hospice movement in the United States and Delhi, Stjernswärd argued that all it had done was to secure expert care for the few who could access it. In contrast, he claimed, the Neighborhood Network model was a big step toward securing universal coverage for pain patients. As for the question of "quality," it was moot if care did not reach most of the patients who needed it. Stjernswärd spoke plainly in his criticism of Gupta's position: "Our colleague does not accept the number of people covered by a program as a measure of its effectiveness and suggests instead the quality of care as the measure (without a numerator). Really? Instead our colleague has an ethical problem with the community approach stating, 'Is it right to offer people something just because there is nothing, or are we duty bound to strive for the best even though we may have to limit the numbers we are caring for in the process'? Really!"[33]

These arguments about the possibilities and limits of community participation are not new to global health. The who formalized the framework of community participation as one of its guiding principles in 1978.[34] It remains a guiding principle in many global health policy proposals such as the un Millennium Development Goals and the World Bank's poverty reduction strategy. T. N. Madan writes of how community participation was taken up in the 1980s in India in the policy recommendations of the Indian Council of Social Science Research, the Indian Council for Medical Research, and the Indian government in its five-year plans.[35] But while the model was unevenly implemented elsewhere in the country, it took deep roots in Kerala.[36] In 1996, the newly elected Left Democratic Front Government in that state launched an ambitious plan to decentralize planning and promote community participation in government.[37] Through this plan, the government handed over direct control of about a third of its planning budget to local councils and municipalities. This devolution of power was a response to years of activism, civil society mobilization, and a slow change in vision within the Communist Party of India. At present, Kerala far surpasses the rest of the country on most indicators of health care quality, even as it continues to struggle with entrenched gender, caste, and class hierarchies.[38] The success of the Kerala model and its success with community participation have attracted international attention, leading to many health care partnerships between organizations such as the WHO and the government of Kerala. Palliative care has been no exception to this Kerala health care story. While the state has only 3 percent of the country's population, a study published in 2008 found that of the 139 points of delivery for palliative care in the country, 83 were based in Kerala.[39] In 2008, the Kerala government consulted with the state's leading palliative care professionals to draft an official state policy regarding the practice. It recognized the NGOs engaged in the work and allocated significant resources to help them extend the model for the entire state. In the practice of palliative care in Kerala, the motives, aims, and aspirations of state and NGO actors have almost become indistinguishable, as the leading NGOs are given broad latitude to define state policy. In stark contrast, the Delhi government took sixteen years to respond to court directives to ease its drug control policies and make oral morphine available to cancer patients. In the meantime, it had taken Cansupport five years to procure its license to distribute morphine.

We see, then, the differential possibilities open to NGOs, vis-à-vis their relation to state governments. Crucially, we also see how the concealment of cancer becomes a matter of policy debate. On the one hand, advocates of the Kerala model argued that state support, education, and capacity building would redress the problem of concealment. Concealment, in this understanding, presented a symptom of a deeper malaise—that of social inequality— and thus was not the primary object of public health intervention. "Awareness" campaigns were proposed as being enough to deal with the problem of an information lack. In contrast, Gupta and Cansupport grappled with the extraeconomic stakes of secrecy, the unpredictable etiologies of stigma, and the centrality of kinship and neighborhood politics in inflecting disclosure and concealment. Reflecting on Cansupport's extensive experience with stories like the ones presented at the beginning of this chapter, Gupta argued that they could not place the responsibility for intervening in this nexus of social relations and illness on those already caught within these fraught social ties.

The Intimacy of Strangers

If in practice Cansupport's workers operated within the norms of concealment around cancer, every year they organized events that staged globally recognized tropes of disclosure and survivorship such as a "Walk for Life," a "Run for the Cure," and so on. These fund-raising events brought together celebrities, politicians, diplomats, and families of staff with groups from schools, corporations, and a range of other professional organizations. However, the gathering intended more directly for the beneficiaries of Cansupport's home-based care was Remembrance Day, a smaller and more somber annual event. Because of the structures of concealment that isolated patients and families, this event was often the only time that Cansupport's clients encountered each other, as well as anyone from the organization apart from the team that visited them. During the month leading up to the Remembrance Day, home-care workers asked family members they had grieved with that year if they were ready for a public voicing of their loss. If the family or a family member expressed interest, the team would then invite them to the event. The year of my fieldwork, the event took place at the India International Center (IIC) in central Delhi. The IIC is one of the country's most elite cultural institutions, set up by the Rockefeller Foundation and the Indian government in the decade following decolonization. Since then, its membership has been restricted to the highest political, cultural, and social class of the capital. Given the class demographic of Cansupport's patient base, most families did not even know of the existence of the IIC, which is located in the middle of Lutyens' Delhi—an area of ten square miles that is named after the colonial architect Edwin Lutyens, who designed it in the early twentieth century. This was a part of the city that Cansupport's patient base would rarely have occasion to visit. While the exclusivity of the place gave a few some pause, most agreed immediately in a show of genuine gratitude for the organization.

Cansupport's fourteenth Remembrance Day began on a chilly winter afternoon on the front lawns of the IIC. The ceremony was punctuated by the release of balloons and a Sufi musical performance, leading to the main draw: testimonies of Cansupport caregivers and patients' families. The first testimony was by a newly recruited home-care doctor who had previously served in the Indian Medical Service wing of the Indian army. He began his testimony with the globally recognizable metaphor of the war against cancer:

> The thing that has struck me the most in working with Cansupport is the team's approach. In the army, we were always told that battles are fought to be won. That perspective might lead us to think that when a patient dies, we lose that battle. But this is a misconception, because as you all have heard, "love conquers all." Now I know when a patient dies, it is not as if we lost the battle. It is a different kind of victory, a different kind of mental resilience, it is a "spiritual victory" both for us [the caregivers] and for you [bereaved families]. When we arrive at a patient's house, I saw something I never saw in my work elsewhere, a happiness that lights up the home. . . . I just want to say that this is not a losing battle, and that victory comes under the maxim—love conquers all. Please pray for me, that I can become a good team member too.

The theme of his speech was to rethink the metaphor of a "war" against cancer: he reframed the war as a striving for resilience in the face of death rather than as an aggressive battle for survival. His call was echoed in almost every testimony that followed, as caregivers reiterated the idea of a shared struggle, of how their personal pain was often resolved through their hope of easing the pain of others. A young man in his thirties articulated this theme from a different point of view:

> My name is Suresh, and I have lost my mother to cancer. I have always been a student of science. We are always taught that it is in science and only science that we place our faith. Two multiplied by two is always four, it is never five. My mother was suffering from a rare cancer called pancreatic cancer; maybe it is very common now. When I confronted it, or I should say, when my family confronted it, we were confused. We didn't know where we were, what was going to happen, there was a dark tunnel in front of us and we were asked to walk through it. And then we landed up in Apollo [a private hospital chain]. [The] rest you can understand what Apollo is, and what goes on there. I saw science lose every day there. That fight continued for three years. For three years, my mother was all right, so I thanked science for extending the years in her life, which meant a lot to my family and me as well. But

the day I found out the doctors had given up, and they said that it was better to take her home, that we realized what we were actually fighting for, that day I understood that science, our friends, life, and hope, all left our side. We could not confront this truth. We had no idea how to break this news to her that she is just going away. . . .

Then a friend called me and told me about "palliative care." I'd never heard about it, it's probably for only the most knowledgeable. Then I called Cansupport. The way she listened, she should train all the call center workers in America. I felt like my pain and my pain only was heard, it was the biggest pain in the world. The next day, imagine our surprise when we found a doctor in our house. She was unlike any doctors. For the first time, we actually *welcomed* a doctor to our house. And she was different. My god what a woman she is. Our house that had been shattered was, for the first time, again a home. We felt for the first time that we were tied together again. Perhaps the pain became common and shared between us. . . . The nurse touched my mother. For many days nobody had touched her, my sister was scared to wash her parts. My wife was hesitant to go near her. I do not have the words to thank her. They taught me that my mom was going away, and how I could say good-bye to her. Cansupport touched my life, and today I have realized it has touched many lives apart from mine. Thank you for calling me to speak.

Suresh echoed the army doctor's critique of scientific hubris and of the use of war as a metaphor for treating cancer. Even as both slipped in and out of using the metaphor themselves, they established their distance from its implications of victory and defeat, reformulating the criteria of victory as the capacity to endure in the face of death. Suresh's testimony also touched on a theme that ran through the day's speeches: what it means to form relations of pain. A middle-aged man, Bhupendra, tearfully described the affective tenor of such a form of relation. While he spoke, the team member could not help but revert to a role of care, placing his hand on Bhupendra's back in a gesture that reverberated their year-long relationship:

We are all in a state that leaves us bereft of words. How do we even express our gratitude to Cansupport? We have lived our lives in pain, and I cannot find the words to describe in words how Cansupport supported us. . . . When they come to our house, we felt like our house, which had been drowned in the darkness of grief, was lit up for a moment. Here, someone has lost a son, someone might have lost their mother, I lost my mother, someone lost a friend, the relation that we have among us, is a relation of pain. And as they say, relations of pain are the strongest relations. No one can tear this relation apart. I remember this line: Where there are relations of pain, what is separation? Those that have faced death are never separated. Our relations are relations of pain, and they will remain for the rest of my life. I had once asked the visiting team about Harmala Gupta. They had told me that she had gone through the same disease, and understood its pain, and had founded this institution to take away this pain. I will always remain tied to Cansupport, and I will never forget you, or the team.

Moments later, Bhupendra's curiosity about the relations of pain found echoes in another testimony:

I do not know what to say, I only know that I have to say, this is the first time after coming to Delhi that I met people who care. I can only recite a poem, I might not remember it correctly, but I must say: "In this concrete jungle, there are houses as far as the eye can see. But as much as I searched, I could not find a human being." Then I met a junior doctor in Lok Nayak Jai Prakash Narayan Hospital [a prominent government hospital in Delhi]. He put his hand on my shoulder and he said, whatever you do, commit this number to your heart, they will stay with you to the end. My uncle was sick. "Uncle" is the wrong word to use, he was not my blood relation, but my father, my mentor, my guru. The day I realized he was my guru was back in 1998. In 1998, my brother's dead body was burning on the pyre and I was crying. He came to me and put his hand on my shoulder and said, this is life, this is the end, which must come to everyone. When I got that number, I thought how does it matter, let me just call it. It was probably just another number. Every medical facility was saying let's diagnose, let's do this, nobody was saying to me you are going to lose your father, your uncle. I just suddenly dialed the number from my mobile. All I said was that I'm at the hospital, I might call you again. I was shocked when four days later, they called *me*, and asked me—how is he? They made the "I" and "you" of this city an "us."

This possibility of forming relations of pain—relations like, but not the same as, relations of blood—was a consistent theme in the day's speeches.[40] A Muslim man described the uninvited nature of this relation, which even as it was forced, opened new possibilities of joy:

Dear friends and elders, my prayers to you. I do not have the words or vocabulary [*alfaz*] to testify to what Cansupport did for us. I can only say, recite this couplet I heard when I was child: "The road to the mosque from my house is far; come, let us make a crying child laugh." Many tried to explain the meaning of this couplet to me, but I only came to realize what it meant when I met Cansupport. We were desperately circling AIIMS for treatment. Everybody here knows what it is like there, the load is so understandably high. We were living our lives downcast and without hope when Cansupport themselves came to us. In a materialistic place like Delhi, where the corrupt propagate their activities, we took it that they were just another of those business-people. Without much expectation, we called them on the phone. But what we experienced then, there are no words with which I can give testimony. I didn't want or seek out this organization, but I am now bound in a relation to them. Just give me a chance, give me a day's notice, and I too want to go with you to serve somebody. Maybe this will bring joy to my father who died. [*Breaking into tears*] I could not be made happier, if for just one day, one hour, I could help become related to someone the way you related to me. The work that you do, I don't think any other kind of work could bring you so much joy. I fold my hands in prayer to you.

Not only patients but also caregivers spoke of the intimacy possible between strangers, at the same time that intimacy was difficult to achieve amid the fraught undertones of kin relations. A counselor who had been with the organization for four years articulated her journey from a professional to a personal relationship with cancer in the following way:

I joined Cansupport four years ago as a counselor. When I started, I did not know that someone in my home would get cancer. In the organization I worked before, people would be cured with medicines. Then I thought, why don't I help those that are more desperate. I came to know of Cansupport through their foundation course. In the beginning I was scared and asked myself, how do I answer all these questions? For example, someone is about to pass, in their terminal stage, and if they ask me—do I have cancer? How am I supposed to say to them—yes, you have cancer. What answer should I give? Shall I die in pain? I didn't know how to answer these questions. When I joined Cansupport, they said you can't answer these questions without training. . . . When I began to learn from Cansupport, I'd share with my father what I had learned. He said to me amazed, this is wonderful work, don't you ever leave this organization. A year later we found out that he had prostate cancer that had spread to the urinary tract. He knew that if I evaded the question, something was serious. He asked me, do I have cancer? I folded his hands in mine, and said yes, you do. He asked then, how long do I have? I said let's go to the doctor and ask. The doctor said you could live for four to five years. He replied, that's a lot, I can live with that. When we got home, he laughed and said, looks like we should call the Cansupport team now. I didn't know what to say. I was sad to make that call, but I was also relieved that the things he could not ask me, he could ask them. When I got home from work, he would tell me how much he had joked and laughed with the team and complained about me to them. I asked then, do you want to go live with your son, would you be happier there? He immediately shook his head and said no, this is where the Cansupport team comes.

Even in the close relation between the counselor and her father, there remained questions that could not be asked or answered. The intimacy of strangers—founded on the safety of distance—allowed for conversations that were too difficult to conduct with even the closest kin.

It is possible to think of the sudden proliferation of speech at the Remembrance Day as a rupture from the ordinary rhythms of Cansupport's work, since with the patient's death, the previously unsayable had suddenly become sayable. At the same time, such an explanation only partially explains the affective texture of the day. Take, for example, Suresh and Bhupendra's surprise, as they were struck by the presence of so many other families that Cansupport had assisted. Their interaction with the organization had been intensely private until this time; it had been structured by the secrecy around the disease, dictating that only a few team members entered their homes, without public markers that would signal their house as home to a cancer patient. To them, and for every other family there, the existence of Cansupport as a large NGO had been background noise to the scenes of care transacted through individual team members. In this world, events such as the Remembrance Day were remarkable because they were striking exceptions to the proximal registers through which Cansupport's practices of care were transacted within homes and families.

But even as they were exceptions to the usual arrangements of care, testimonies folded back into the intimate tableaux of care of the months gone by. The testimony of a young woman in her early twenties best captures this continued knotting of care and grief. After she took the stage to speak about her grief in losing her father, she choked up in heaving sobs within the first few words of her prepared script. She interrupted her tears to say to herself and to the others present, "I have to do this," trying to begin reading again. A voice from the audience shouted in support: "Be brave, speak, be brave." Immediately, three counselors from the Cansupport staff rushed to her side, holding her while she struggled through the rest of her words. It was a bodily posture they were all accustomed to, as they had sat silently many times with patients for hours on their beds, holding patients and families. The lines between a public testimony from one to many anonymous others fell away to reveal the intimate engagements at the heart of Cansupport's affective work. Minutes later, the tableau would be almost replicated, with another daughter who struggled to speak, again bringing an unscripted onrush of counselors. Minutes later, this intimate configuration would reassemble around a mother who had lost her thirteen-year-old child. If the Remembrance Day intended to collectivize grief, these recurring gestures instead commemorated the everyday, individuated form of care and support. Even at this moment of its most public articulation, grief folded back into its most private, intimate form.

Writing about grief in the context of infant deaths in rural India, Sarah Pinto tells a hauntingly beautiful story that bears repeating here: "At a group singing for a birthday, a woman is passed the drum. She hands it back and says, 'No, since the death of my son I do not sing.' Women nod. The drum is passed to another singer."[41] Reflecting on this moment, Pinto asks: "What then are the ways that death can—and cannot—be named in the spaces just at the edge of institutional certainty, the ways that stories open up an unsteady normality?" This shifting movement between institutional intervention and its manifest intimacies was at stake in the unsteadiness of the testimonies offered over the day. The naming of grief was the explicit script of the event, but at the same time, the difficulties of its narrativizing always pushed against the script, obscuring any certainty that these profound losses could be cathartically released. The Remembrance Day, then, was certainly a departure from the usual reticence toward speech about cancer. The event brought families closest to the institution that cared for them, allowing for a circumspect and scripted public narrativizing of grief. In all this, the event produced a genre of recognizable speech—the trope of testimony directed at a collective audience bound by shared experiences of suffering. At the same time, the event reflected the more intimate context of Cansupport's everyday work—within neighborhoods and homes, in small rooms and at bedsides.

The moments that scripts fell apart revealed the difficulty in scaling up and translating these intimate and bounded relations of pain to more abstract registers of something like communal bereavement across families and institutions. As I understand it, these unscripted repetitions of intimate scenes of care among a few strangers returned families and teams to the intimate and fraught arrangements of sociality within which the disease appeared and unfolded.

Experiments with Relations

In the introduction, I alluded to how psychologists and anesthesiologists interested in palliative cancer care mobilize a putatively Indian capacity for resilience and transcendence as a method to cope with the distress brought about by the disease. I develop this idea more fully in chapter 3. Here, I want to gesture to how the binary between West and East guides another dominant research problem in the literature on the psychological aspects of cancer—the problem of denial and concealment and how they inflect psychiatric distress. For example, several studies over the last three decades examined whether terminal prognoses were communicated to families and patients.[42] Consistently, these studies found that most patients in India were kept in the dark about their prognoses by family members; estimates of this number ranged from 40 to 80 percent. Most such studies hypothesized that the difference might be one of an "individualist" Western culture that privileged patient autonomy, as opposed to a "collectivist" Indian culture where illness knowledge lived with families rather than with individual patients.[43] If ethical norms of autonomy demand the communication of diagnoses in the West, in the "collectivist" East words were not the provenance of individuals, but collectively, of families. And if the "West" has learned to speak and prognosticate openly, it was because of its culture of individual autonomy that privileges transparent communication. Analogous research argued that "denial" might be understood as positive coping, one that might be incorporated rather than vilified in the Indian therapeutic setting.[44] Such studies often contradict each other. Several studies suggested that denial in India enabled psychological coping, while others argued it contributed to psychiatric morbidity, anxiety, and depression.[45] A broad metastudy concluded that denial was best understood as a "dynamic" concept, one that needed to be considered in relation to families and social relations.[46] What I find interesting about these studies is how they go against the grain of received public health understandings that equate the lack of explicit communication about diagnosis with biomedical noncompliance and bioethical wrongdoing. At the beginning of this chapter, I described how the entrenchment of bioethical norms of autonomy obscures the realities of biomedical practice, where the patient's "right to know" is, at best, a distant normative aspiration. As the more nuanced of these psycho-oncology studies recognize, the contexts and effects of denial are far more varied than they first appear, and not always correlational with either a quest for or refusal of well-being.

Yet, if these psycho-oncology studies argue for the importance of understanding denial in a "collectivist Indian" context, my work here rejects such broad cultural explanations of concealment, offering instead more proximal and intimate motivations. Within the same neighborhoods, concealments of diagnoses meant different things for different people and carried vastly disparate consequences. For some, it could evidence transactions of care. For others, it was a strategy to preserve life in response to hostile circumstances. Delving into everyday worlds of the management of illness disclosures and nondisclosures, my work here aims to unravel the binary set up between a knowledge of diagnosis and its absence. In doctor-patient communication, the "knowledge" of illness was not something that was simply transacted from one to another; as in the case of the patient with which I began this chapter, most knew much more than they were explicitly told. Similarly, subsequent concealments and nondisclosures by patients and families were rarely about hiding the "truth" of a diagnosis. Instead, they revealed intricate choreographies of care and danger where certain things were said to some and not others, at certain times, and in certain places. The ecology of concealment was then much more complex than just whether the patient knew or did not know. Even as this binary—knowledge or denial—preoccupies public health and psycho-oncology, I suggest that it is the wrong framing. Shifting the problematic from knowledge to speech opens for analysis the work of speech in managing the social reverberations of a cancer diagnosis. As speech, the dynamic movement between concealments and disclosures evidences careful relational work. Concealment and disclosure evidence experiments in social relations, of how to best live with or alongside a cancer diagnosis. While there might be some truth to prior writings that suggest that nondisclosures show a desire to escape the disease's stigma, my work here resists framing stigma as a set of easily identifiable cultural beliefs diffused through a cultural environment.

Instead, my aim here has been to understand the dangers and desires around nondisclosure as something far more intimately relational. Speech and nonspeech about cancer evidenced a dynamic negotiation with families and neighborhoods, within which each patient grappled with a different problematic of the stakes and effects of concealment and revelation. The Remembrance Day event was striking precisely because of the power of these intimate and proximal registers. Even as the event sought to collectivize grief, the everyday register of the organization's work insistently reasserted itself. The circumspect arrangements of speech and nonspeech, enacted within the porous privacy of homes, were a reminder and remainder even in this most public of events. At the same time, acknowledgments of the disease suffused the day's proceedings. Coming together in a part of Delhi slightly removed from such an immediacy of fraught proximal space afforded the possibility of collective testimony, a genre of speech whose stakes within homes and neighborhoods were far more variable, requiring a different care and caution. In all its variability in these more everyday spaces, speech or nonspeech about cancer resisted reduction. Its motivations were irreducible to typologies of cultural beliefs or stigmas, or to formalization as a "positive" or "negative" coping mechanism. To the contrary, they evidenced the variability of how my interlocutors grappled with the fraying and reknitting of social relations, enacted in these instances through a circumspection about words.

2

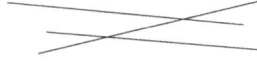

CANCER CONJUGALITY

I did not intend to pay particular attention to conjugality when I began accompanying the cancer care NGO Cansupport on home-care visits. When I first started fieldwork, my questions were about state neglect and abandonment, and I had expected to find patients focusing on those concerns. However, in many of these home-care visits, I found my attention drawn to dynamics of care, love, and neglect within marriages. This was not accidental: spouses were the first line of support for many of the cancer patients we visited. But even within this relation, I began to focus on instances in which husbands were diagnosed with cancer. Although Cansupport visited equal numbers of men and women, I was drawn to this particular intersection of conjugality and cancer because of a recurring ethnographic pattern.[1] As scholars of kinship in India have noted, wives in North Indian family arrangements are often rendered vulnerable because they live in affinal homes, often without recourse to the support of natal kin.[2] In the context of this virilocal vulnerability, wives are often subject to abuse from in-laws and husbands. In her ethnography of poor women in Delhi, Claire Natalie Snell-Rood documents how her interlocutors survived these conditions of structured vulnerability by making distinctions between what they could or could not control, accepting that they could shape "what was in their hands."[3] These circumscribed possibilities of well-being also meant that women often swallowed the knowledge of the harms inflicted on them, maintaining and sustaining relations with violent husbands.[4] Thus, acceptance and reconciliation become a normative horizon, so strong that even domestic violence counseling interventions and women-led marriage arbitration centers encourage a "politics of livability," teaching women to live with and through kinship norms.[5] And even as public discourse charts the rise of "chosen" marriages or shifting customs, for women across many contexts in North India, marriage remains the durable basis for social legibility and citizenship.[6]

In this chapter I explore how in such situations of structured vulnerability, the texture of care extended by wives to husbands with cancer grew out of these deep-rooted conjugal asymmetries. For the first time, husbands found themselves confined to their homes, in contrast to the relative freedom they enjoyed previously. This curtailment was sometimes the result of physical debility, but it also often occurred because the disease's stigma led men to isolate themselves from networks of kin and neighbors. Cancer concentrated the time and space of the conjugal pair, problematizing the relation in new and sharper ways. If maintaining families and the everyday life and health of households was often normatively understood as the responsibility of women, cancer created further responsibilities of care and obligation. At the same time, these deepened responsibilities opened subtle possibilities of inhabiting these norms of care and obligation differently, giving circumspect voice to histories of buried violence—even if for a brief while. Thus, in the dynamics of conjugality after a cancer diagnosis, it often became impossible for me to sift between care and violence: their paths ran through each other, as husbands and wives lived on in sites of prior violence, enacting new kinds of disregard all while sustaining each other's possibilities of life. In her work on the politics of conjugality, Elizabeth Povinelli asks, "Which forms of intimate dependency count as freedom and which count as undue social constraint?"[7] My focus in this chapter is this entanglement of freedom and constraint, of partial speech and secrecy, and of marital disruption and reconciliation in the shadow of cancer.

Love Withheld

On a warm afternoon after the monsoons and before the beginning of winter, I accompanied a doctor, a nurse, and a counselor from Cansupport to an East Delhi neighborhood. The household we visited comprised a married couple in their forties, Shyamlal and Deepa. They lived in a small home they owned with Shyamlal's parents. Shyamlal had been diagnosed with lung cancer about eight months prior to our visit. As we entered, I noticed the counselor taking in the arrangement of furniture in the room. Through my months of home visits with the team, I had learned to watch for this diagnostic glance. The counselor saw that Shyamlal's and Deepa's woven wood beds were both in the same room, but apart and perpendicular to each other. For her, the placement of beds was a reliable clue to the arrangements of intimacy within a home. Shyamlal's bed was pushed up against the side of the room, and he lay with his face pressed up against the wall, unwilling to turn and greet us. This sign of visible annoyance was rare in my visits with the team, and even rarer where the NGO was the only source of licit morphine as an analgesic. Even though India is the world's largest producer of licit opium, narcotics laws restrict it to less than 1 percent of the country's cancer patients. Cansupport was one of the few sources of licit morphine for cancer patients in Delhi. But here, the problem was not of drug access: Shyamlal's pain had resisted high doses of opioid painkillers. Considering this failure, the counselor shifted her attention to matters more social than physiological—sensing that perhaps marital conflict had become part of the etiology of Shyamlal's intractable pain.

Shyamlal had increasingly isolated himself from social contact. As discussed in the previous chapter, concealment was a widespread coping practice among cancer patients and families I encountered in Delhi. Upon learning of the diagnosis, neighbors often do more harm than help. Some grieve and lament patients who have not yet died. Others query kin to discover past histories of moral disrepair that might have caused the disease. Still others recount the pain of others they have watched die. Yet Shyamlal was pushing away not only unwelcome neighbors but even his daughter, with whom he had always been close. She called him on the phone every day, but he almost always refused to speak to her. When they last spoke, he told her that Deepa—his wife—was trying to kill him by changing the dosages of his medicines. The immediate cause for our visit this day was an escalation in his pain. Deepa complained that he had cried out through the night, waking the family and antagonizing the neighbors with whom they shared a thin wall.

The team's visits had settled into a predictable pattern over the past month, and today was no exception. After the doctor and nurse went over details about dosage, symptoms, and schedule, Deepa took hold of the conversation. With repetitive compulsion, each week she narrated different threads of a story of three decades of marital abuse. Each time she would say this was the first time she had spoken of this history to strangers. A major element in this narrative was her description of three affairs that Shyamlal had not even really cared to hide. Deepa hinted that partly because of these betrayals, they had stopped sleeping together about fifteen years ago. As she detailed his unfaithfulness, Shyamlal would often draw closer to the wall, sometimes breaking into groans to drown out her voice. At other times, he would speak directly to the team—as if Deepa were not there—and accuse her of lying. And at yet other times, he would address Deepa and demand renewed conjugal intimacy, begging her to consider that he only had a few months left to live. In turn, Deepa would respond to the team and not him: "I can only give him medicine, I cannot even sit on the same bed as him anymore."

Over time, Deepa's narrative revealed deeper cracks in their relationship. Her natal kin lived in another city. Early in her marriage she had considered involving her mother to help mitigate the abuse she experienced, but she had kept her family in the dark, not wanting to "burden" them with the knowledge of her husband's violent behavior. In these vulnerable circumstances, her parents-in-law had tried to force her to accept a bigamous arrangement. They justified it to her as the family's age-old *riwaaz* (tradition). Although polygyny is illegal according to the Hindu Marriage Act, scholars have documented the continuance of the practice.[8] Deepa had refused Shyamlal taking a second wife, recognizing that she might become even further marginalized within an already hostile household. She told us she might have considered it if she could not deliver male progeny, but she had produced both a son and a daughter and stood firm on the grounds of her reproductive success. Yet, her refusal to give in had earned her violent retribution from her affinal household, whose members had all beaten her in the last decades. She ended one of these visits by reciting a couplet: "Apne se bachke raho, paraye se khatra nahin / vishvasghat ussi se ho sakta hain, jispe vishvas ho" (Beware of your own, there is no danger from others / you can only lose your faith in those you might have once trusted). At another meeting, she had told the counselor that Shyamlal had continued hitting her even after receiving his diagnosis. It was only in the last month or two that he had become too weak to continue.

Their daughter visited from time to time, but their son was a persona non grata in the family. From the counselor, I gathered he was addicted to inhalants and heroin. The counselor had pieced together that Shyamlal had thrown him out of the house a few years earlier. Over the last few years, Shyamlal had turned his attention to his financially unsuccessful younger brother. He had arranged a marriage for him and helped him rent a home in a nearby neighborhood. But after Shyamlal's diagnosis, his brother had stopped visiting or talking to him. The counselor I was visiting with had tried to mend this relational fracture. After much coaxing, Shyamlal agreed to let them call and talk to his brother. We heard later that, shamed by strangers, the brother and his wife paid a visit to Shyamlal and Deepa, but this did not lead to a lasting reconciliation. Now, partly because Shyamlal was estranged from his male kin and progeny—from both brother and son—and partly because he was so dependent on Deepa for care, her position had shifted subtly within their home. Remarkably, he had agreed to sign over the deed to the house they lived in to her, despite his parents' objections. In a context where property is most often transacted along patrilineal lines, removing property from the domain of his own male kin was a late gesture toward mending at least one of his several broken relationships.

Concerned with Shyamlal's recalcitrant pain, the team urged Deepa to swallow some of her anger against him. As described in the previous chapter, the Cansupport workers I was with were committed to treating pain as both a physical and a social concern. They were sure that if the couple could reconcile their differences, Shyamlal's pain would subside, and he would be able to die a peaceful death. When I later expressed my discomfort about this tack to the counselor, she replied that they had a single mandate: to ease the suffering of the patient's last days. Deepa's reactions to this nudge toward reconciliation were shifting and mixed. She had grown close to the team and, by her own account, treasured their visits. They gave her an opportunity to speak and come to terms with her husband's impending death on her terms. But over time, as Shyamlal's illness progressed, gestures toward intimacy took the place of cathartic accusations. If in the team's first visits she would at most hold her husband's hand while he was in pain, in their later visits they would often find him resting his head on her lap. Yet, she never came around to joining the two beds, nor did she give in to Shyamlal's demands for intimacy; his protestations on this count continued. But the subtle shifts in tone and gesture had an effect on Shyamlal. As the team had predicted, he found real relief from his pain, and they were able to cut his morphine dose in half.

What might we make of the team's intervention into kinship and conjugality while treating cancer pain? I do not want to judge Deepa's experiments with speech and silence as leading to either catharsis or further damage. For decades of her marriage, Deepa had kept silent about Shyamlal's many betrayals and violations. Her silence had been a way for her to cope with her affinal hostility. But now, ever so slightly, Shyamlal's diagnosis had allowed for the possibility of speech. At the same time, to say Shyamlal's cancer had tipped the scales and opened new possibilities of recovery for Deepa would be going too far. Deepa's response had been a careful and dynamic arrangement of circumspect speech and voluble silence. Her strategies of living alongside Shyamlal's death are evocative of descriptions in Clara Han's work in Chile on everyday care and obligations and relations that are lived, embodied, and experimented with.[9] Han writes of how even in times of extreme duress, individuals remain caught within webs of social relations and continue to awaken to new dynamics of social connections and disconnections. She writes of these times as not normless, or outside the norm, but as experiments with life. The analysis of these experiments of care that emerges in Han's work shows the deep intertwining of care and violence in the work of living on in the aftermath of medical crisis. Thinking of Deepa's strategies as shifting experiments with norms helps me understand how she both achieved and lost a sense of well-being in proximity to her husband's death.

Words in the Wind

At the beginning of a visit to a home in West Delhi, the team parked our car near a large open sewer and made the rest of the journey on foot. After a short walk, we arrived at a small convenience store. Suresh, the owner of the store, had been diagnosed with laryngeal cancer about two years earlier. As far as the doctor on our team could tell from Suresh's reports, his cancer was in remission after six months of chemotherapy. When we arrived for this visit, Suresh motioned to us to go to his house above the store—laryngeal cancer had robbed him of speech. He gestured that he would close the store and join us soon. Upstairs, Suresh's wife, Sunita, broke down in tears before he arrived, telling us, "He beats us all; he isn't himself after he's finished his bottle at night." While she spoke, one of her two sons walked in; he looked to be in his mid-twenties. They took turns telling us that two nights ago, Suresh had picked up a metal pipe and threatened to beat them all with it. The two sons had managed to restrain Suresh and tie him down to the bed. The son looked upset as he said that he never imagined he would raise his arms against his own father. The counselor intervened, aiming to tackle Suresh's alcohol addiction. "What do you think is leading him to drink? What is it that seems to be making him angry? Do you think it might be the stress of the illness?" Mother and son replied almost in unison: no, it is not the illness, he has always been like this, it is just habit [aadat], there is no cause. The counselor asked, "Why not talk to the treating oncologist at Guru Tegh

Bahadur [the public hospital where Suresh was getting treatment] and get him admitted for de-addiction during his next visit?" Mother and son were incredulous at this suggestion. Sunita explained, "The doctor is moody. If he finds out about the addiction, he'll stop treating him. He'll cut the phone if we even say the word 'addiction.'" For most families, effective cancer treatment is scarce. To negotiate the many forms of triage in public oncology facilities, patients must make themselves out to be ideal candidates. This involves trying to hide anything—including alcoholism—that might signal future noncompliance.

After spending two hours talking to Sunita and their son, we walked down again through the store, making our way out onto the street. Suresh had come upstairs during that time, but sensing the tone of the conversation, he made a sound of disapproval and returned to the store. When we finally left the house, Suresh waved to us that he would follow us to the car. We waited for him to join us, and he arrived in a few minutes. Seeing my fieldwork notebook in my hand, he gestured to ask if he could borrow it. He turned the pages to the end and started writing. After every few sentences, he tore the page, handed it to us, took it back after we read it, crumpled it up in a ball, and threw it into the wind, in the direction of the sewer.

Suresh's story contradicted his wife's version of events. He wanted to convince us he had been sober for years and that his daughter's death a few months earlier had forced him back to drink. The counselor told me later that Suresh's daughter had been married about a year ago and had indeed died a few months later in her affinal home. The family suspected dowry murder but were hesitant to initiate a long police and judicial process. Suresh then wrote that his daughter's death had opened his eyes to the plight of his new daughter-in-law. He explained that his wife had found their son his bride, and that she was both five years older and five inches taller than their son. Their son had agreed to this marriage, but he begrudged his bride both her years and her height and hardly ever allowed her out of the home. Then, Suresh wrote that Sunita and their sons resented him not because he drank but because he advocated for his daughter-in-law. He rejected his wife and son's story that he assaulted them; in fact, he said, it was the other way around. The violence the neighbors heard was from when he tried to protect his daughter-in-law when Sunita and their son attacked her. Later, the counselor and nurse talked about how they had seen the daughter-in-law looking distressed in previous visits. Suresh then gathered the crumpled words that the wind had not carried into the sewer and stuffed them in his pockets.

It is not for me to adjudicate the truth of either Suresh's or Sunita's narrative. Rather, I want to locate how this speech and silence folded into broken kinship worlds. When asked whether cancer had contributed to Suresh's addiction and violence, Sunita had contested that framing, suggesting instead that it was aadat. The word *aadat* translates to both "habit" and "addiction," and its double valence is telling. When asked by the counselor, Sunita refused to identify cancer as the rationale for Suresh's addiction and violence. At another visit, she confirmed Suresh's claim that he had been sober for about two years before his diagnosis. Importantly, then, while Suresh and Sunita disagreed on the what and why of the violence between them, neither placed its weight on cancer. Recall that Suresh had offered his daughter's death, not his own disease, as the proximate cause for his return to addiction. Both Suresh and Sunita folded the disease within the everyday give-and-take of violence and addiction.

In thinking about the unstable relation between disease and habit (aadat), I am reminded of Zoë Wool's and Veena Das's delineations of the critical and the normal.[10] Both warn against drawing clean, self-evident lines between the ordinary and the catastrophic, focusing our attention instead on their dynamic entanglement. The diagnosis of cancer did not wrench Suresh out of the everyday. Instead, prior and new failures of social relations—between son and father, wife and husband, affinal and natal kin—haunted his life with the disease. The form of this haunting was not that of an inversion of the ordinary. It was not as if the patriarch's cancer overturned ordinary arrangements of silence, speech, and gendered violence. If Deepa's experimentations with life blurred the lines between harm and well-being, a similar incoherence was at stake here. Threatened with cancer, Suresh had been brought close to death and robbed of speech. But while norms and ordinary arrangements of violence and speech bent under the pressure of disease, they did not break. As much as Suresh and Sunita disagreed on its form, they agreed on the fact of the enduring vulnerability of women to affinal violence. As for who occupied the position of the witness, that too was not a settled question. Neither was it self-evident whom the intersection of violence and disease had silenced, and whom it had rendered voluble. We saw how as Suresh threw his words to the wind, the wind carried some to the water but returned others to his feet. I can find no better image to describe the weaving together of critical illness and the fragile norms within which they appear and retreat.

The Promise of Self-Harm

The Cansupport team and I were struggling to find a house we were visiting for the first time. Walking through the narrow lanes of a housing settlement in the southern edge of the city, we asked for directions and were guided toward a plot of land littered with construction materials and equipment. "Construction" is often a precarious time in Delhi; thefts of material and illegal land grabs are always an imminent threat before built structures are occupied. Charandas, the sixty-year-old patient we were visiting, had come into some money through the sale of his agricultural land in Kishangarh, a nearby newly developing area. He bought this plot with that money and, with his wife, Lalita, moved into a room that was part of the ongoing construction. Together, they kept vigil over the construction site. However, right from the beginning of our conversation, I saw how this promise of a stable future in brick and mortar was haunted by the instability of an embittered marital past. Charandas had been diagnosed with pharyngeal cancer about three years earlier. He had stopped visiting his oncologist after a year of treatment. He had not kept his medical records, and his prognosis remained unclear to us. His first words of greeting to our team were: "I stay awake from one to four o'clock at night, every night. All I think of is suicide, the only thing that is left is the *action* [in English] itself." The table in front of him was littered with *beedis* (local cigarettes), but this was not his only addiction. He was a heavy drinker, and after his diagnosis he developed a dependence on narcotics and, most recently, a generic form of Spasmolin—a drug that slows the activities of the brain and nervous system. Charandas and Lalita sat on two different beds, at perpendicular angles as far from each other as possible within the space of the room.

In her conversation with the Cansupport counselor with whom I was visiting, Lalita confessed a narrative of thirty-five years of marital conflict. Willing at first to speak only to the counselor, Lalita called her aside, and they talked for almost an hour in whispers on Lalita's bed. The doctor and I continued to talk to Charandas. Later, the counselor told me in broad strokes the themes that recurred in many of the families I visited: addiction, domestic violence, and hints of long histories of the husbands' extramarital affairs. Later visits would reveal that this couple's history of marital discord had been exacerbated by a string of recent familial events. Their young, unmarried daughter had worked part-time at a Hindi-language call center in the nearby township of Gurgaon. A few months ago, she had not returned from work. They later found out that she had eloped with a Muslim man from her workplace. This contravention of intrareligious kinship norms had brought shame to their Hindu family. Charandas complained, "This happens in upper- and lower-class families. For a middle-class family like ours, this means ruin." Lalita elaborated further, "She has more or less killed us. But how could she have done otherwise? All she saw between me and my husband [was] his mistreatment of me. We failed to raise her the right way." After a prolonged period of silence, two days before our visit, the daughter had called and informed them that she and her lover had run away to Pune. Her two brothers had sworn violent revenge on both sister and brother-in-law if they ever returned to Delhi.[11] Lalita said, "They hate her for what she has done to us and want nothing to do with her ever again." Lalita wanted nothing to do with her husband, blaming him for their present troubles, including losing a daughter and losing their ability to give her away in a marriage of their choosing. The counselor tried to reiterate a familiar theme in the affinal politics of Indian kinship, saying, "Girl children are anyway never your own. They always belong to someone else [affinal kin]." Lalita countered, "But not in this way, we were never able to give her away." Charandas's response was equally accusatory: "Why do you only think of the past? You're killing me now and our future. Let this cancer take me, I don't care about living, if living is like this, with her." The doctor continued to speak to Charandas, asking, "Do you get out and get fresh air in the day?" Charandas countered, "How can I show my face in this neighborhood? I used to pass the time by standing out in the street. Now I cannot look at how the neighbors look at me." The anxiety about respect and shame in the neighborhood continued to poison the marriage in the present, bringing the ongoing difficulties of a thirty-five-year marital history to the surface. Yet, unable to share intimacy, they continued to build a dwelling.

The course of the disease and the course of the decaying kinship biography ran together. The breaks in kinship ties had slowly chipped away at Charandas's will to live. He had stopped treatment, and developed and exacerbated his addictions to nicotine, narcotics, and painkillers. The team would say later that it was miraculous that while so many others fought desperately for the last months of their lives, Charandas's willful acts of self-harm had not visibly debilitated him. As Lalita would tell the counselor, the illness had placed a burden of care and responsibility on her. Her response took the form of a constant vigil; she had nursed her husband through the most difficult periods of his illness. Yet, like Deepa, she had found herself unable to mingle care with love. Charandas's will to live depended on the mingling of the two. He said simply in response: "I can't live without you." His cancer certainly lent weight to his utterance. Yet, a history of domestic violence, addiction, and extramarital affairs haunted his words, undermining this late gesture toward reconciliation. In this case too, the experience of critical illness disturbed social mechanisms through which gender and intimate power hierarchies were muted, allowing histories of violence to rise to the surface. But it was not just cancer that had disrupted their everyday negotiations of living together; it was also their daughter's elopement. The co-incidence of both kinship and disease opened the possibility of public expressions of the past to cancer care workers. The possibility of Charandas and Lalita's future was staked on this house, but the past made living on difficult.

It was in this context that Charandas enacted and threatened self-harm. As he told it, his increasing dependence on substances resulted from the betrayals *he* had suffered: first by his daughter's elopement, and then by his wife's inability to reconcile with their past for the sake of their present. By his account, he had lost his will to live because of them, and not because of the onslaught of cancer. Because we did not know his prognosis, it was difficult for us to sift through his narrative claims. The team remarked on his apparent good health, comparing him to other patients under their care. Yet, they also knew the appearance of health could be deceptive. But, if I move past the desire for certainty about his etiology, something other than the relation between cause and effect becomes clearer. As a performative gesture of self-sacrifice, Charandas was trying to recover a position of authority within the household, a position that had come into question after his diagnosis. In the presence of strangers, Lalita had laid bare his failings as a husband and father. Bearing in mind Deepa and Shyamlal's story from earlier in this chapter, I understand Charandas's suicidal discourse as having more to do with the gendered asymmetries of power than as revealing of how the disease had exhausted his will to live. Bearing witness near death is not an ethical act of achieving narrative closure to a life, but a battle for recognition. These testimonies to strangers reveal much about the shifting dynamics of who can bear witness, how (through speech or silence), and to what (past or present betrayals). Thus, bearing witness to death is not only a gendered act but also revelatory of the shifting grounds of gender asymmetries in the shadow of critical illness.

The stories so far of conjugal violence and intimacies have described couples in which both members were alive at the time of my fieldwork. The next story describes how past betrayals continue to poison the future even after a spouse's death, inflecting accusations and threats of self-harm. One of the more affluent patients I visited with Cansupport lived in a two-story home.

The family we visited had prospered in the neighborhood as the provisions store they owned had benefited from the area's rising prices and incomes. In the last few years, they had bought two more stores close to the first. The patient we were visiting was an elderly woman, Mohinibi, who had been diagnosed with ovarian cancer more than a year earlier. She smiled at us as we entered; the team had been visiting the family for several months now and had become fond of Mohinibi. Her high morphine dosage left her sedated and groggy. After the usual greetings, Mohinibi declared that the next time we would visit, she would no longer be around. I took this to mean that she had accepted her advanced cancer, but quickly realized that she meant something different. Mohinibi's husband had died a few years earlier and had bequeathed this property to the four sons in the household but left nothing for Mohinibi or their daughter. She described both her loneliness after losing her husband and her anger at how he had left her with nothing. (We never had occasion to meet her daughter because she worked during the days we visited, but we knew she was unmarried.) A claim for recognition was implicit in Mohinibi's anger. She suggested that she had suffered much in her marriage, and that this elision from her husband's will—even though it was conventional—was the last slight, and more than she could bear. A few months before this visit, she had threatened to immolate herself in front of her family. The threat had alarmed her sons and was the reason they had first called the Cansupport team to their home.

To our visiting eyes, her sons seemed devoted to her care, and their neighbors told us they were the pictures of filial piety. During our visits, Mohinibi would engage the team in cheerful conversation, at the same time as she would describe new ways she had thought of to bring about her own death. The newest method she wanted to tell the team about was to drown herself in the nearby Yamuna river. To dissuade her, the counselor expressed concern that given how the Delhi police responded to such suicides, the real brunt of these injuries would fall on her sons. She suggested to Mohinibi that they would be taken into custody for alleged complicity or force, and in jail, they would languish for years under the slow judicial system. The counselor then asked Mohinibi if she loved her sons. Her answer was an emphatic yes. The counselor countered with why, then, did she want to see them in jail after her death? This conversation had played out earlier in a similar vein, but this time Mohinibi was prepared with a response: she declared that she would explain it all in a suicide note. The counselor countered that the police would assume that she had written the note under duress.

The tenor of these negotiations is hard to describe. The reciprocal affectionate humor and care in these exchanges belied their seriousness. While the counselor was worried about repercussions for the family, she was also invested in protecting Mohinibi from self-harm. In other visits, Mohinibi's repeated suicidal threats elicited the team's stories about the troubles of other families. A few months prior, the team's counselor had visited an aging husband and wife. The husband had been diagnosed with cancer, and the wife had taken the diagnosis as an opportunity to take revenge for years of marital abuse. Years before the diagnosis, her husband had abandoned her after she gave birth to their son. He had returned five years later, and she had reluctantly taken him back. Now, after his diagnosis, he was completely dependent on his wife for his daily care and hospital visits. Echoing a theme that runs through this chapter, she declared that she would care for him, but could not mingle that care with love. The idiom of her dissatisfaction took shape through the modalities of care. For example, she would boil his glucose water to an uncomfortable temperature before giving it to him to drink. He would reciprocate by putting her cutlery into the blender, or by mixing jaggery (unrefined sugar) in her dough, making it impossible for her to knead it into bread. After months of such minor aggressions, he threatened to commit suicide and leave a note that would blame his wife for his death. His wife had put an end to these threats by warning him of the implications this would have for their son. She had asked: Did he want to see their only child give up his education and spend his life trying to get his mother out of jail? The counselor's experience with this couple had given her clues on how to prevent Mohinibi from inflicting further harm on herself. She understood Mohinibi's threats of suicide for what they were: claims of recognition for herself and for her daughter to those around her—her sons and their families. Instead of denying those claims, she sought to counterpose them with Mohinibi's enduring obligation and affection toward her sons.

Failures of Recognition

Several scholars of Indian medicine and social life have borrowed an emic category—*sevā*—finding in it conceptual tools to parse the violence and care that run through Indian familial life.[12] For example, Lawrence Cohen and Sarah Lamb use the term to understand the work of intergenerational care.[13] When focusing on the care from sons to parents, both Cohen and Lamb describe sevā as a marker of power, overtly of the elder being served, but covertly of the increasing power of sons as their father's strength declines. Yet, both describe how the promise of sevā as a transfer point of power remains provisional; old age continues to have a voice and to demand authority, while children's sevā is always partial and falls short of its ideal. In this subtle balancing act of familial authority, excessive demands of recognition risk being labeled as deviance. Particularly clear in Cohen's description, an excess of voice sometimes masquerades as psychiatric madness, a failure of "adjustment" in old age that threatens the stability of intergenerational power.

I think of sevā here not in relation to intergenerational care but as a transfer point of voice through which conjugality is negotiated in times of illness. As a relational action enacting a shift of authority from the receiver to the giver, sevā helps parse some scenes I have described. To understand sevā requires sensitivity to the complex and shifting conjugation of speech and silence in marriages. In conjugal care as it appears here, the wife's sevā is both a form of intimate care and a subtle enactment of partial critique. Withholding love from care—or at least making certain to distinguish the two—motivated the narratives of several of my interlocutors, including Deepa. Yet, the insistence of Cansupport workers on mingling care with love, especially at the end of a patriarch's life, entailed a new form of adjustment, reconciliation, and acceptance. In her work on domestic violence interventions, Julia Kowalski writes of how counselors operationalized sevā as a framework and context within which they offered women advice.[14] Kowalski argues that instead of emphasizing a liberal conception of autonomy and independence as a solution, they emphasized interdependent relations of sevā, working within ideologies of patriarchal kinship to offer a subtle reordering, rather than escape, from household violence. In the absence of robust frameworks for the assertion of legal rights, this compromise—in which they substituted "women's rights" for more secure kin-based dependence—was the best solution at hand. Much in the way Kowalski describes, the counselors I worked with also encouraged conciliation over rupture. For example, in emphasizing the reintroduction of love in the work of sevā, they too sought to work within and through kinship norms.

At the same time, the crisis of cancer focused the time and space of the conjugal pair in ways that are subtly different from other contexts of conciliatory interventions. Kowalski describes how counselors intervened in kinship by shifting the focus of disagreements away from the conjugal pair to disorder in other kin relationships, such as those between the wives of elder and younger brothers, that were more amenable to change. But in the shadow of cancer, kin both within and outside the household sometimes became distant and reluctant to take part in the daily work of care. In other cases, even when wider kin networks were available as a source of support, wives were expected to take on the daily and demanding work of caring for weakened husbands. At the same time, prior asymmetries in mobility came to be limited by the debility brought on by disease. Condensing past violence, present disagreements, and impossible futures, the time of cancer focused attention on conjugality in ways from which there was no escape. Importantly, this is not to say that conjugality came to stand apart from and outside wider kin relations. As in my description of Mohinibi's case, transactions of neglect, violence, and care often seeped through and across the boundaries between marital and intergenerational relations, while tracking gender lines. While conducting fieldwork, I chanced upon a Hindi play about cancer—*Behatar Hain Maut* (A desire for death)—that precisely dramatizes this potential juxtaposition of intra- and intergenerational sevā in the time of critical illness.

A Desire for Death

The play takes place in the aftermath of the cancer diagnosis of Narendra Mohan—a sixty-five-year-old man who lives with his wife, Ramadevi, his unmarried daughter, Neelima, and his two sons. Narendra is beset with unbearable cancer pain, which breaks into the play's script as half-blank pages, incomplete words, and onomatopoeic syllables. As Narendra's pain heightens, he describes it as his closest kin. Yet, in the play's action, Narendra's pain takes a backseat to an unfolding family drama. The characters of the play are taken from a stock of kinship tropes that are the staple of Indian family dramas: two sons (one dutiful and the other profligate), a devoted daughter, and mistreated elders in a time of social change. In the second half of the play, the profligate son marries a wife who is equally uncaring toward his father, and together they lay claim to parts of the house the father had occupied. In this new arrangement, the father is relegated to a corner of the house where he no longer feels able to entertain guests, and he becomes increasingly isolated. While Narendra has few expectations of his profligate son, he is disappointed by how his devoted son also feels exhausted from providing care. Tired of suspending his own life for the sake of his father, the once devoted son marries and moves away to a different house. With both sons absconding from their responsibilities, Neelima is left alone to care for her father. In contravention of the ideal of sevā, but close to its practice, women are left to bear the burden of care without the privilege of a transference of intergenerational authority. Neelima gives up hope of marrying, as her own romantic interest tires of waiting for her and moves to another city.

Toward the end of the play, the mise-en-scène shifts—away from the intimate space of the home to a courtroom where we find Neelima and Narendra begging the judge to allow his assisted suicide and his release from the unbearable pain of his cancer. Neelima has heard that the rich have access to "clinical death," and she demands that the poor also be given this right to *iccha-mrityu* (self-willed death). But Neelima's eruption into public speech is short-lived. After only two pages, she is returned to silence. From then on, she appears only in relief to the volubility of reporters, kin, lawyers, religious leaders, and doctors who decry her plea, ask for her arrest, and point to her as the perfect manifestation of *kalyug*—the mythic time of social decay. Finally, only on the last page of the script, Neelima breaks both her silence and the fourth wall. She does this to declare that she had spoken not with the expectation of relief but in the certainty of the failure of her speech to be heard. This draws fresh ridicule from the chorus, who see her now as a hysteric, as having lost her sanity. The play ends with her plaintive lamentation to her dead mother: "I cannot bear this responsibility over life and death any longer, mother—please come, please come and take this responsibility back. Please take it back."

What I find remarkable about this play is its return to the theme of women bearing the responsibility of witnessing and lamenting. Neelima laments the pain of her yet alive father, abandoned in a zone between life and death. But, in her lament, she only briefly faces the judge or the journalist—as they stand in for public order. In the closing scene, she directs her lamentation instead to her dead mother. Ramadevi's death, which occurs halfway through the play, happens off-stage and is only evoked by Narendra's monologue in the middle of the play. His wife's death occasions his thoughts on the intimacy between life and death, and how death carries life around like a cat carries its young, with her teeth grasping the nape of the kitten's neck. We are never told the circumstances of her death; rather, the reader is left to surmise that it had something to do with the exhaustion of care. I understand Neelima's lament, then, not just as a critique of an unjust social order—personified by the chorus—but also as an invocation of female kinship in shared suffering. In her final scene, she reaches out across the threshold of life to her mother, whose presence and silence haunt the play. She testifies to this silence that she is bound to inherit. But rather than giving speech to the failure of the social order, she testifies to its arrangement of recognition and misrecognition, within which she knows in advance she will never be heard. There is, then, a double structure to her witnessing: she testifies not only to her father's cancer but also to her inability to fulfill her role as a witness through which his death can be rendered good. As in the stories of the patients presented in this chapter, Neelima's activity lies somewhere between silence and speech, between representation and expression. In her inability to shift legal and familial norms, she captures how these norms structure the force of recognition, within which the pain of her father, the silence of her mother, and her own disempowerment are fated for the shadows.

As disease enters kinship worlds, it articulates with the past, present, and future in unpredictable ways, folding into preexisting arrangements of betrayal and reconciliation. It does not overturn and rupture social worlds, as much as it comes to be diffused throughout an existing social field, all the while absorbing, augmenting, or hardening prior vulnerabilities. In these instances of North Indian kinship, the disease shifted the capacity of husbands and wives to inflict and absorb violence. The debilitating experience of cancer often confined husbands within their homes and, for the first time, made explicit their dependence on the gendered work of everyday care. Consequently, these subtle shifts opened cracks in the domestic world that allowed for long histories of violence and betrayal to seep through and become speech. At the same time, cancer did not invert existing norms of speech and silence around gender, allowing women the possibility of free expression they did not previously enjoy. They continued to inhabit the vulnerable space of affinal homes where speech always carried with it the possibility of future harm. In such a world, speech and silence often followed the other's tracks, one taking the place of the other, as time and necessities shaped their possibilities.

A Turn to Myth

In the last two chapters of this book, I shift my method from face-to-face ethnography to readings of aesthetic accounts of cancer. Doing so helps me sharpen my ethnographic descriptions, as I put the neat resolutions of aesthetic accounts in relief against the unresolved ethical dilemmas that pervade my ethnography. Here, I pause for a moment to think about Indian mythology as a bridge between the ethnographic and the aesthetic. I do so because Indian mythology has proved an especially generative ground for scholars of gender and sexuality in South Asia. As Sarah Pinto suggests, myths need not appear in ethnographic accounts only in relation to the interpretive work they do for our "real" subjects. In her work, she asks whether we—as readers and storytellers—can welcome mythological figures into our work as imaginative grounds of our own writing and thinking.[15] Similarly,

Veena Das writes of how she draws simultaneously from both literature and ethnography as figures of thought to expand what we take as a shared conceptual vocabulary.[16] Thus, anthropologists of South Asia move between the mythic and the present in ways that evoke a richness of ethical potentiality, or, as Michael Fischer calls it, their structural plenitude.[17] In doing so, they move between their own interpretive frames and those of their subjects. Drawing from this work, I place my ethnographic stories in this chapter adjacent to Indian mythology. Doing so thickens the conceptual vocabulary with which I parse the gendering of witnessing, lamentation, and speech around cancer.

Pinto finds that, broadly, Indian epics allow women two interrelated positions in response to violation: righteous speech or a turning into stone.[18] But in certain moments, Pinto suggests that women can do both—deliver an indictment *and* disappear into silence. Every ethnographic figure who appears in this chapter inhabits this taut dynamic between speech and silence, between indictment and the swallowing of past betrayals. Recall, for instance, how Deepa linked speech and silence to the possibilities of her endurance. At the same time, she found ways of expressing how the world she inhabited had often turned on her. In her experiments with endurance, she was always cognizant of the damage her invocations of past violence could bring to her life in the present. Deepa's experiments remind me of the mythic figure of Gandhari—a woman who must also negotiate the fraught ethical world in which she finds herself. In the Mahabharata, Gandhari is the mother of two groups of warring cousins. She is married to a blind king and is famous for wearing a lifelong blindfold as a sign of devotion to him. While this gesture might be read as an act of subservience, in the epic Gandhari gained so much power through this self-denial that she developed a second sight. And it was through this second sight that she became the most powerful witness to the carnage of the battlefield at Kurukshetra, in the war between her sons and their cousins. In the Mahabharata, it is Gandhari, and Gandhari only, who can eclipse the corruption of recognition and the fragmentation of grief. Through Gandhari, the myth clarifies that sight is no easy path to unobstructed vision; rather, her blindness is one of the few moments of ethical clarity in the epic. Yet, the form of this clarity is not certainty—in the Mahabharata, there are no easy answers about what constitutes virtue and evil. Those who promise the clearest vision of morality are often the figures who fall the furthest short of their goals. Synthesizing these mythic lessons, Pinto parses Gandhari's act of witnessing not as clarification of right and wrong but as an observation on the failure of recognition.[19] I too find remarkable this structure of Gandhari as a witness, and how her testimony juxtaposes sight and blindness, fragmentation and wholeness, speech and silence. Deepa reminds me of Gandhari, and Gandhari reminds me of Deepa, in their threading together of restraint and indictment.

Gandhari is not alone in exposing ethical uncertainty in the Indian epics. In times when certainties of good and bad deaths come undone, and when women lament not to resolve death but to mourn ethical violations, Veena Das is reminded of Draupadi.[20] In the Mahabharata, Draupadi is married to the righteous Pandava brothers, the enemies of Gandhari's sons at the battle of Kurukshetra. But for all the Pandavas' claims to morality, they gamble Draupadi away in a rigged game of dice. As a result, Draupadi is brought into the gambling hall, and the winners of the game begin to disrobe her. At the moment of her disrobing, however, she appeals to Krishna, who, impressed by her commitment to dharma, turns her sari into an unending length of cloth. This scene is iconic in India's cultural imagination and has been rendered in many visual and written forms.

In Das's description, Draupadi negotiates a difficult line between testimony and silence, expressing the violation of her disrobing by not shedding her soiled robes for fourteen years. And it is not only through her body that Draupadi offers an indictment. Before her disrobing, she throws the hall of men into jeopardy by speaking and calling their adherence to dharma into question. What draws me to Draupadi here is that, like Gandhari, her act of bearing witness to violation is enacted through a conjugation of speech and silence. Gandhari delivers an indictment through her blindness and returns to silence. Similarly, Draupadi offers an indictment through speech, only to find the possibilities of speech again taken away. It is these momentary eruptions into speech that give weight to these women's subsequent silence. And only when we place their silence and speech next to each other can we can hear the force of their indictment. As Das puts it, Draupadi's questioning will continue to haunt the rest of the epic, as a reminder of how ethics once became mute in the face of a question asked by a woman. "Even if the war will be won, the self and all forms of relatedness will become frayed, if not lost."[21] I can think of no better way to parse the complex conjugations of Sunita's, Deepa's, and Lalita's speech with their silence, as they negotiated the fraying of their social relations in the shadow of cancer.

If Draupadi and Gandhari are two of the most prominent figures in the Indian mythic imagination of lamentation, Antigone—in her lamentation for her brother—stands in a similar place of witnessing in the European imagination.[22] In Sophocles's play, Antigone breaks the law of the king (Creon) by transgressing his decree that her brother not be buried or mourned. Some scholars read her as a transgressive figure who defies Creon and bears witness to the unjustness of the law of the state. In other readings, in her refusal to bend to Creon, she stands as a witness to the unjustness of the social order within which she is bound. It is enlightening to place that canonical figure in the European imagination against her much humbler counterpart whom I discussed here—Neelima. Both Neelima and Antigone rail against a social order, gendered male, that blocks their kin from achieving a proper death. But if Antigone's lament is directed at the king, standing in for a just order, Neelima's is directed at her dead mother, invoking the possibility, already eclipsed, of a shared female kinship. Unlike Antigone, she does not ascend to the status of a fully formed subject through this act of transgressive speech. Instead, she descends back to silence and joins her mother in the shadows of the play.

Finally, then, I find the complexity of these Indian myths a useful conceptual framework because of their essential ambivalence about the redemptive possibilities of speech. The figures of Gandhari and Draupadi open the possibility of the ethical in acts one might otherwise understand as a defeat. These acts include the confrontation of violence with silence, and a desire to retrench the self in one's own world rather than a desire to escape it. Most powerfully, these myths show how accusatory speech carries with it a double indictment when it folds back into silence: an indictment of a world that is not made for the speaker to thrive, as well as the structures of recognition that do not allow certain kinds of speech to become legible grounds for action.

3

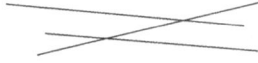

RESEARCHING PAIN, PRACTICING EMPATHY

The word "cancer" hides more than it reveals. Scientists and doctors often correct its unqualified usage, pointing out that cancer is not just one disease, and that contemporary fears about its ubiquity are based on this misunderstanding. Rather, cancer is really an ensemble of specializations, modes of diagnosis, and kinds of treatments. So, when I naively began fieldwork at the All India Institute of Medical Science (AIIMS) hoping to study cancer, it quickly became clear I would have to focus my inquiries much more narrowly and concretely. What were the specific practices I would examine within this constellation of specialties, practitioners, and patients that constituted cancer care in this specific hospital? For example, studying the medical physics or radiology units would direct me toward practices of imaging and testing. Working in the medical or surgical oncology divisions would focus my attention on diagnostic and therapeutic interventions. Or following the cancer registry would turn my attention to the relation between demographics and health policy. Such units and departments make up most cancer hospitals worldwide, and each would have made for its own research site.

However, my attention was drawn to a corner of the cancer hospital that is not globally ubiquitous—a unit staffed by anesthesiologists specializing in cancer pain and dedicated to palliative care. The presence of this unit surprised me partly because palliative care is globally still quite a nascent biomedical field. The first hospital-based palliative care units emerged in the late 1980s and 1990s in Europe and the United States. But even as the field has continued to grow in the twenty-first century, the specialization remains peripheral to supposedly more urgent oncological modalities—radiation, chemotherapy, and surgery. For example, at the time of my fieldwork, less than a fourth of the major cancer hospitals in the United States reserved beds for palliative care as was done at AIIMS.[1] And if palliative care is uneven in places like the United States, it is almost absent in most of the global south. A 234-country survey conducted during the time of my fieldwork found that about a third had no palliative care services of any kind.[2]

The presence of an advanced palliative care unit at the cancer ward at AIIMS—staffed with experts and allocating beds to palliative care—reflects how, as the country's leading hospital, AIIMS can claim an exceptional amount of government resources. Its annual budget of about $226 million is around 4 percent of the national health budget.[3] At the same time, the cancer hospital was dedicating expertise to palliative care in ways that far surpassed what was being done at many of its peer institutions elsewhere in the world. Even in the most well-resourced hospitals in the global north, the field of palliative care still draws its practitioners from undervalued, low-prestige specializations such as social work, counseling, nursing, and mental health. At AIIMS, the core staff of the palliative care ward were practitioners at the opposite end of the biomedical hierarchy: anesthesiology.[4] Further, as Sarah Pinto and Cecilia Van Hollen describe, anesthesiologists are a rare commodity in Indian public health.[5] Instead, they remain caught within a conventional ordering of public health priorities—urgent and life-saving treatments first, care and concern for "symptoms" such as cancer pain later. At the cancer hospital, my interest was thus drawn to this puzzling presence of a team of dedicated anesthesiologists, all transacting palliative care in a hospital struggling to provide timely conventional therapies.

In this chapter, then, I track the emergence of cancer pain as a central preoccupation at the cancer hospital at AIIMS. Usually considered by public health and biomedicine as a symptom and not an urgent subject for intervention, how did pain become such a central concern here? I found that palliative care specialists understood that to treat pain, they had to treat the social worlds within which pain takes shape. In conversations, medical journals, and practice, they defined "total" cancer pain—a condition that was simultaneously social, spiritual, psychological, and physical. Here, tracking cancer pain as a subject of research and intervention, I come to understand the pathways through which these specialists translated social, spiritual, and psychological distress into physical pain, and vice versa. Further, I find that the possibilities of treating pain understood in this way were staked on specialists' understandings of "culturally appropriate" modes of empathy and humane practice. While tracking cancer pain, then, I also trace these responsive visions of empathy. Thus, two questions guide this chapter: What does cancer pain, in its intensifications and obfuscations, teach us about the infrastructures of care within which it ebbs and flows? And what have been the felicities and failures of the modes of empathy that have emerged in response?

Total Cancer Pain

The AIIMS campus sprawls under one of the busiest traffic intersections in New Delhi—a crisscrossing layer of overpasses referred to as the AIIMS flyovers. A few high-profile patients, ministers, and bureaucrats reach the institute by driving along these overpasses; others take buses or autorickshaws or use the subway system. Some have traveled from the edges of the ever-expanding metropolis, while others have made their way from more distant parts of the country on the subsidized national railway system. At the main gate, hawkers sell food and illicit brokers peddle hospital forms to patients and their attendants. Many of their customers have camped outside the walls of the institute for weeks. The well-guarded entrance gate bottlenecks a steady stream of ambulances, cars, pedestrians, and staff. Beyond the entrance, in contrast to this crowded space, the 233-acre hospital campus is lined with trees and dotted with open gardens. This contrast reflects the founding vision of the institute, whose first buildings were constructed in the heady first decade after Indian independence as part of Jawaharlal Nehru's plan for the new nation-state. Nehru's dream was that along with the nearby Indian Institute of Technology, AIIMS would produce a class of Indians insulated within elite centers of excellence.[6] These scientists and researchers would be free from government interference and the uncertainties of social change. Thus unencumbered, they would work on the native Indian subject as a resource to educate and cultivate. Srirupa Roy describes these spaces as nation-statist heterotopias, imagined as unmarked by identities and interests.[7] Others shared Nehru's vision. Brought to India as a scientific consultant in 1943, the British Nobel laureate Archibald Hill recommended that "a great All India Medical center should be established, an 'Indian Johns Hopkins' staffed in all departments by the ablest people everywhere."[8] In 1946, a committee led by the Indian civil servant Sir Joseph Bhore took Hill's advice and gave AIIMS its name and institutional structure.[9]

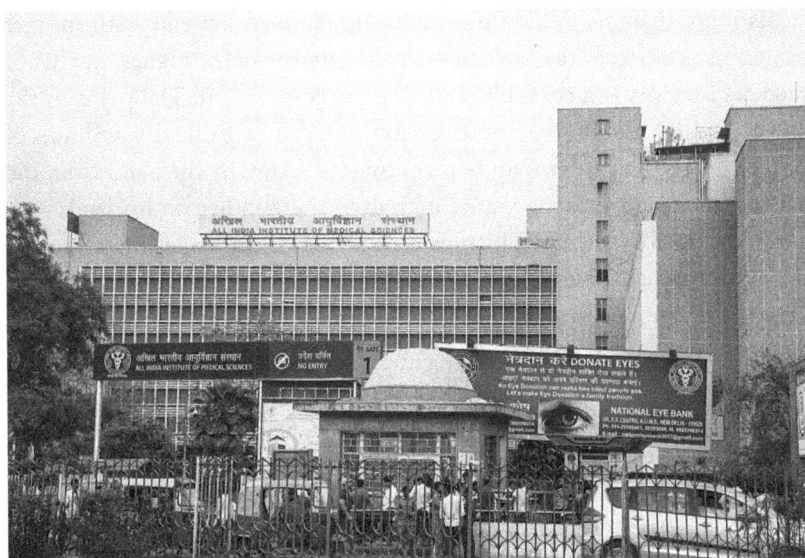

FIGURE 3.1 The All India Institute of Medical Sciences (AIIMS). Photo by Javed Sultan.

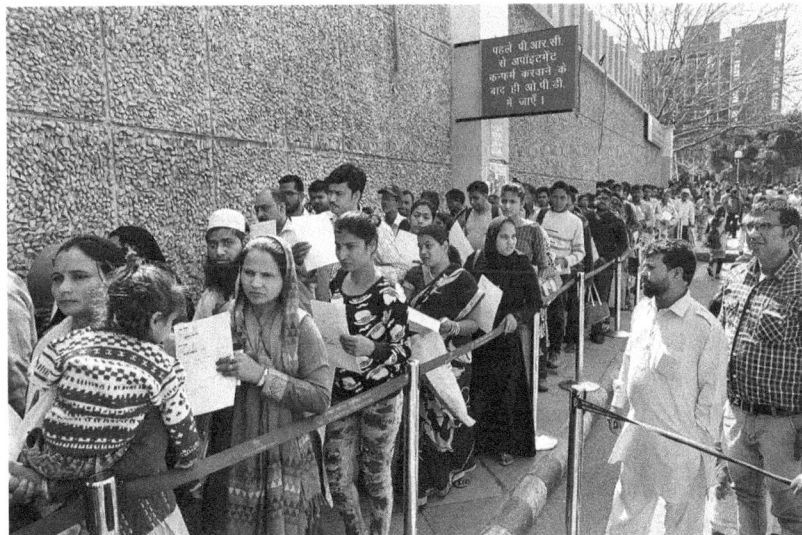

FIGURE 3.2 Patients queued outside the gates at AIIMS. Photo by Sushil Kumar / *Hindustan Times*.

In the present, the heterotopic fantasy of a space insulated from social chaos falls away as soon as one enters its gate.[10] The institute estimates it treats more than 3.5 million outpatients every year. Patients with meager economic resources are drawn here by the promise of the highest quality of medical services at a cost subsidized by the government. The paths to the superspecialty buildings evidence relationships of care under conditions of duress: a child, no older than ten, guiding his father by the hand from the subway to the entrance; a young man carrying another on his back with a practiced effortlessness. The most debilitated lie on makeshift stretchers outside buildings. Before they encounter medical staff, they will have to negotiate the fixers who surround the building. The wait time for tests performed within AIIMS can be a few months; these fixers arrange to have patients' tests done at nearby diagnostic centers, charging them a higher fee. Some will help patients jump the queue or, for a larger fee, even secure hospital beds. Security guards with whistles patrol the buildings and manage crowds. Mostly, their whistles warn errant visitors away from restricted spaces. Sometimes, they deliver warnings, clearing a space for emergency patients rolled on stretchers along potholed roads. AIIMS is more the debris and ruin of a heterotopic historical vision than its practical realization.[11]

During my fieldwork in 2012, I found the cancer hospital exemplary of the paradoxical juxtaposition of care and duress at AIIMS. Called the B. R. Ambedkar Institute Rotary Cancer Hospital, it is one of twenty-seven state-accredited regional cancer centers for all of India. Many patients travel here over long distances across North India for treatment. In part, they are drawn to the center by the reputation of the country's flagship public hospital within which it is situated. To meet with a specialist, patients and their families queued inside and then outside the building in the early hours of the morning. The first queue led to rooms that housed patient records. New patients had a new file recorded, and returning patients registered their arrival; then, both sets of patients joined longer queues that led to three outpatient rooms. The process of queuing took several hours, culminating in a short ten- to fifteen-minute consultation with a specialist. The most debilitated lay on stretchers along the passageways; others stood, to not lose their place. The outpatient meeting rooms were some of the busiest and most chaotic spaces at AIIMS. During prearranged clinic hours, teams of doctors would arrive, jostling past patients to make their way into the rooms. Once past the crowds, they would seat themselves around two or three small tables while a staff member brought them the day's patient files. During each scheduled four-hour outpatient time, three or four doctors would meet with

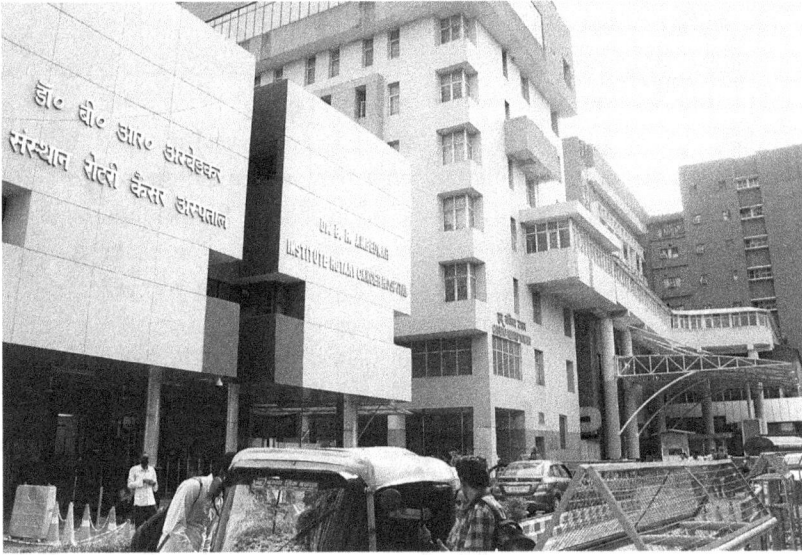

FIGURE 3.3 The B. R. Ambedkar Institute Rotary Cancer Hospital at AIIMS.
Photo by Javed Sultan.

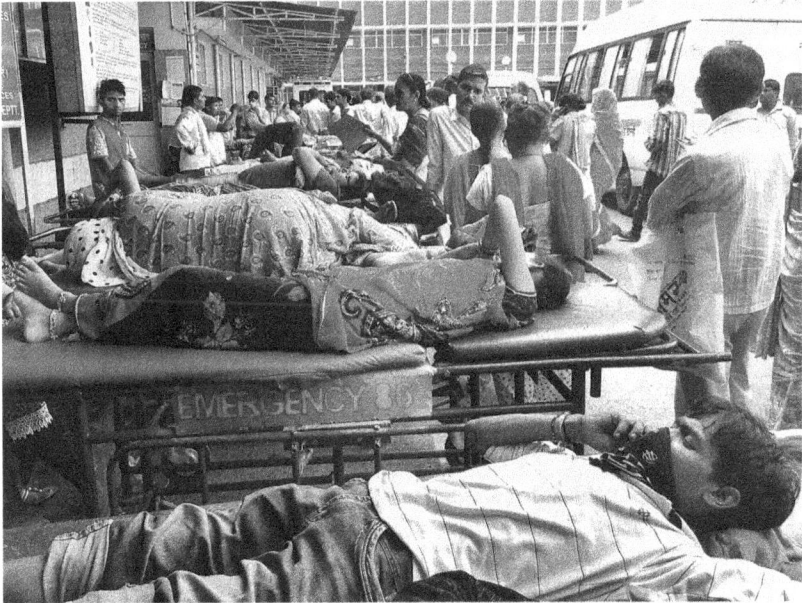

FIGURE 3.4 Patients waiting on cots outside the emergency ward at AIIMS.
Photo by Saumya Khandelwal / *Hindustan Times*.

more than one hundred patients. This included glancing over patient records, recording new data, conducting diagnoses, prescribing medicines, scheduling tests, and communicating prognoses. Here, as Julie Livingston observed in Botswana, the form of triage was multilayered.[12] An independent journalistic investigation into AIIMS in 2011 revealed that getting an appointment for an MRI could take anywhere from a month to a year and that a CAT scan has a waiting period of more than four months.[13] As for curative interventions, surgeries for malignant tumors could take up to six months, while patients with benign tumors waited nearly two years.

Under these conditions of infrastructural pressure, pain often accompanies cancer. To elaborate, for patients diagnosed with certain types of cancer, pain is inescapable. Tumors may compress the spinal cord, damage nerves, press upon organs, or spread to bones. At times, pain is also an outcome of cancer's highly debilitating treatments—surgery, chemotherapy, and radiation. But for all its variations, one predictor of the presence of cancer pain is the stage to which the disease has progressed: it is twice as likely that a patient will experience moderate to severe pain if their cancer is advanced.[14] It is no surprise, then, that in India, where patients are almost always diagnosed at late stages of disease progression, pain is an overwhelming part of cancer. Such a strong association of pain with cancer is inevitable in other parts of the world too, where infrastructural conditions do not support timely diagnosis. For example, global health researchers describe a "pain gap" between the global north and global south, captured succinctly by a Lancet Commission report which indicated that in 2015, 80 percent of the 25.5 million people who died with need of and without access to palliative care were from lower- and middle-income countries.[15] It also found that only twenty countries in the world had integrated pain specializations into their public health systems.[16]

While global health experts have only recently described a global "cancer pain epidemic," palliative care practitioners in Delhi have been actively responding to the condition for more than two decades. My first clues to the practices that have cohered at AIIMS appeared in a conversation with Dr. Abha, an anesthesiology resident in the palliative care unit: "When I was fresh out of medical school, I used to look at a patient and say if you have lung cancer, you should have pain in the chest, and nowhere else."[17] The complex pathways, etiologies, and somatosensory frameworks of cancer pain require specialized medical training; these concerns were not part of the traditional training of an Indian anesthesiologist. Dr. Abha laughed and added something that every resident told me during my fieldwork: "You know, practicing palliative care, you really shift in your orientation. You begin, or at least try, to think of pain from the patient's perspective, or even the family's. You begin to see *through the patient's eyes*" (emphasis added). This orientation that Dr. Abha pointed to—of seeing "through the patient's eyes"—was the mantra of pain therapeutics at AIIMS; I would hear it again and again in conversations with other residents, at training sessions for doctors in different parts of the city, and in weekly staff group meetings. Of course, the encouragement to cultivate an empathetic orientation in medicine extended beyond the specificity of palliative care at AIIMS. I could find similar exhortations—"to adopt the patient's perspective," "to share the patient's pain"—in palliative care textbooks published in North America and Europe. However, hearing it repeatedly, I wondered about the specificity of empathy in this pain clinic, and the distinct orientation that residents were urged and able to cultivate *here*.

Dr. Abha and I were talking in the room in the anesthesiology unit that housed the old research computers I was working on. The room doubled as the residents' makeshift office space, where they took breaks for meals, conducted impromptu meetings, and discussed difficult cases. It was just a few feet wide and long and contained a small sofa and dusty piles of old, discarded patient files. While I queried an institute database for a project I was collaborating on with the residents, Dr. Abha described a battle between the head of the palliative care unit—Dr. Nigam—and the hospital bureaucracy. "It took Dr. Nigam ten years to even get us this small room and the six-bed inpatient unit. Earlier, we just had an OPD [an outpatient department], and soon realized that if we were to do any meaningful work, we needed to admit patients! She fought for years, and they finally gave us the six-bed ward. It's not much, but it is at least a start." The struggle for space and resources reflected a broader disciplinary struggle to have cancer pain recognized as a syndrome in its own right, and for palliative cancer care to be recognized as a specialty with its own standing. Finishing her lunch, Dr. Abha good-humoredly pointed around and told me, "Imagine, at first we didn't even have any space to show our families around when they would come to visit us at work."

The emergence of palliative care both at AIIMS and in Delhi has much to do with the charismatic head of the anesthesiology department. Dr. Nigam began her career in 1991 at a small municipal hospital in Bombay. In 1999, she was hired as an assistant professor at AIIMS, and by the time of my fieldwork in 2011–12, she had risen through the ranks to a full professorship. She was also a founding member and editor of the *Indian Journal of Pal-*

liative Care and served on several governmental committees on regulating pain management. She has been responsible for introducing the specialty to this flagship government institution's teaching curricula and therapeutic practice. AIIMS remains one of the few medical teaching institutions in the country that recognize palliative care as a specialty. At the time of writing, it offers both a doctoral program that allows students to specialize in palliative medicine and a postdoctoral fellowship leading to a further subspecialization in onco-anesthesia. Dr. Nigam had also campaigned for renaming and upgrading the palliative care unit as the Department of Onco-Anesthesia. "Onco-anesthesia" was a hyphenated neologism I had never heard before I worked at the ward. It was only a year later, while scouring medical publications, that I found the word in the title of an article in an international anesthesiology journal that prospectively called for such a future subspecialty.[18] At AIIMS, Dr. Nigam was anticipating this future, and her pioneering work had not gone unnoticed. Her office desk was lined with several international awards, including a prestigious one from the International Association for the Study of Pain. She was involved with World Health Organization (WHO) initiatives to develop shared pain management expertise across developing countries in Africa, South Asia, and Southeast Asia.

But for all her international recognition, the achievements she took the most pride in were the young residents she trained to specialize in the emerging discipline. Given the specialization's relative lack of prestige, this had been no easy task. At the time she entered the field, government funding for cancer care was already plagued with problems. A senior oncologist recalled how the visit of a foreign dignitary in 1998 occasioned a paint job worth 400,000 rupees, while his request for the sterilization of the unit's toilets was dismissed as too expensive. At the time, he went on, one of the CAT scanners at the institute had been in need of repair since 1991, the inpatient units lacked air conditioners, and the outpatient waiting rooms did not even have fans for relief from the heat of the Delhi summer. It was within these infrastructural challenges that Dr. Nigam had started a new palliative care ward, secured a space for outpatient meetings, and set up the residents' office.

Within these infrastructural limits, Dr. Nigam and her teams of residents worked tirelessly to sketch out the contours of cancer pain as a research and therapeutic object. She was an exacting mentor, demanding that the residents not only keep up with an exhausting patient load but also complete a monthly quota of publishable research. During my time there, I would design and execute two collaborative clinical research projects with the residents, one of which was published, and the other used as the starting point for new projects.[19] The published article was a clinical audit of the pain ward. The second aimed to redesign the clinic's pain assessment procedures, paying special attention to factors understood as nonbiological or "psychosocial" indicators of distress. Both projects immersed me in the complex world of clinical research and diagnostic questionnaires concerning pain.

While similar questionnaires used elsewhere in the world have been standardized to ensure quick quantification and comparison, an examination of the institute's questionnaire revealed a different story. First, I found that given the constraints of time, questions understood as "psychological" and "social" were often left unanswered by examining doctors. Second, even for those that were filled in, the overall design hindered standardized quantification contributing to an overall score. Third, a study conducted at the pain clinic seven years earlier by clinical psychology researchers had discovered high incidences of "depression" and "anxiety" among cancer patients.[20] However, in the outpatient questionnaires I surveyed, such conditions were rarely reported. The recommendations we made at the conclusion of the study demanded more attention to depression and anxiety during interviews. I also suggested in the paper that we adopt a research instrument validated in Kerala.[21] This instrument—called the Distress Inventory of Cancer—was the only one I found in India that related socioeconomic conditions to psychological distress. Its authors highlighted the importance of socioeconomic standing, educational background, and the quality of medical infrastructure in easing or increasing psychological pain. In our collaborative paper, I wrote that given the vulnerabilities of the institute's patient population, this diagnostic instrument would be more sensitive to psychosocial distress.

While our collaborative work was well received, I soon realized that research had a more complicated role to play in the institute's setting. In a meeting about future collaborations, I asked the residents if they knew when our recently completed research would be translated into practice. The residents met my question with equivocation. Finally, one of the more senior residents, Dr. Arjun, demurred by asking me to help him administer the existing pain questionnaire during the next outpatient clinic. As I helped him do so, it quickly became clear that the heavy patient load made the administration of most global instruments exceedingly difficult, if not impossible. We were scheduled to spend four hours in the outpatient clinic. Administering the pain questionnaire to the first patient, I watched the clock run up to fifteen minutes before I finished. Looking at the queue, I saw at least forty patients impatiently waiting in line for Dr. Arjun. Meanwhile, his lesson taught, Dr. Arjun had abandoned the questionnaire for his usual mode of outpatient examination. While I had been administering the questionnaire, he was talking to an elderly woman, who was flanked on either side by her two sons. She had her medical records with her, which showed she had advanced chondrosarcoma—a type of bone cancer. When Dr. Arjun asked for the X-rays, one of her sons replied that they were with another doctor. This response was not uncommon at the pain clinic. It usually meant one of three things—the tests were lost; the tests were indeed held by a private physician who did not want the patient to seek treatment elsewhere; or the patient and/or family mistrusted the tests or else were withholding the results, hoping to get a favorable second opinion. Dr. Arjun asked the woman directly to describe her pain. She said it throbbed like a gas flame and was becoming more constant. A month ago, it was worse at night, keeping her husband and daughter-in-law awake. Now, she could not really tell much of a difference between night and day. Dr. Arjun nodded in response and turned his attention to a lump close to the woman's left knee. The sons interrupted, never once mentioning the word "cancer," calling the lump a *soojan* (swelling). Dr. Arjun quietened them with a look and began to feel his way around the lump. With just two fingers, he pushed and probed, asking at short intervals: "Does it hurt here? And now? And here?" He nodded and gently felt around the edges of the growth. When the woman tensed up, Dr. Arjun reminded her to relax and trust him. While continuing to sense his way, he asked her to stretch her knee and to stop where it was uncomfortable. He also asked which position she found the most restful. He then returned to the focal point of the lump, this time pressing more firmly and judging the woman's discomfort. Satisfied with his examination, he looked back once again at the sheet of paper they had brought, as if to confirm what he had just felt. Dr. Arjun asked the sons where they lived and worked; I knew from prior exams that this was his way of ascertaining what drugs they could afford. Determining from their responses that they were neither wealthy nor extremely poor, he prescribed a cocktail of generic morphine, an antidepressant, an anti-inflammatory painkiller, and an anticonvulsant. As the woman left, I asked Dr. Arjun why he had not asked for further tests. He replied that asking for further tests would lessen the chances of their returning to the pain clinic, and that his touch examination had helped him confirm that the tumor had metastasized rapidly. He guessed, too, that the oncologist had understood that curative treatment would be futile. Finally, he recognized that the sons had kept the diagnosis from their mother, but that she too knew all about her condition. How Dr. Arjun would gather all this from the conversation and exam remains somewhat of a mystery to me; pressing him further did not yield new insight. Instead, he shrugged and said it was "experience" that had taught him pain diagnosis, not just textbooks. Mercifully, he did not mention the pain questionnaire.

Administering even the shortest versions of global cancer pain questionnaires, let alone finding the time to score and record them, had been a lost cause. Instead, Dr. Arjun's lesson was an education in tacit knowledge—a familiar anthropological preoccupation I had almost lost sight of. In his canonical work, Michael Polanyi made the simple assertion that we can know more than we can tell.[22] He deepened this insight by suggesting that processes of scientific formalization often threatened to destroy tacit knowledge gained through proximal, personal, and bodily encounters. One might think of testing and quantifying as precisely such moments of formalization. The tactility of the knowledge that Dr. Arjun possessed was not easily amenable to quantification—either as a research model or as a questionnaire. In itself, this resistance of the practical to abstraction is not surprising. I want to point out here the particularity of the relation of the tacit and the explicit. Pain practice took place in conditions of infrastructural pressure where even the conduct of research itself is a luxury. It relied on habit, experience, and tactility. It engaged the sensory and experiential in ways that opened therapeutic conversations, relationships, and possibilities. Pain questionnaires, in contrast, engaged the body more distally. Rather than play a significant role in guiding practice, they often helped gather data for research. In what follows, I delve deeper into this tension between practice and research and between the proximal and the distal. On the one hand, practice engaged the somatosensory in ways that allowed for certain modes of empathy to cohere. On the other, pain research helped establish the grounds on which palliative care could grow as a biomedical field. Cancer pain—as both a therapeutic and an epistemological subject—cohered in this push and pull between research and practice.

The Metaphysics of Research

The possibilities and limits of cancer pain research in India first presented themselves to me during the annual conference of the Indian Association for Pain and Palliative Care at Kolkata in 2012. Dr. Nigam and the residents at AIIMS were among the event's headliners. I had traveled to the conference to present some of my early ethnographic work while also hoping to speak with leading cancer pain specialists from regions outside Delhi. It quickly became clear at the conference that cancer pain research in India was at a stage where some of its most basic vocabularies were still uncertain. Unsatisfied with the applicability of pain research developed in the United States, several participants spoke about the need to develop indigenous cancer pain questionnaires. One presentation included an anecdote that described the difficulty of indigenizing an American pain questionnaire that asked whether the patient ever experienced the sensation of "butterflies in the stomach." For a while, the discomfort of several patients when asked that question perplexed the doctors who were administering this questionnaire. Only after several weeks did they realize that the phrase "butterflies in the stomach" had elicited concerns about meat eating among vegetarian patients. Interrupting the laughter that followed this anecdote, a senior doctor from South India raised a question about a specific American diagnostic instrument he had been considering for use at his hospital. In responding to this question from the floor, one panelist wondered in passing about how that doctor could afford the high copyright pricing on that instrument. The uncomfortable conversations that followed soon revealed that the doctor had not known that such tools were under copyright in the first place. The murmurs that went around the conference hall revealed that he was not alone. Already, it seemed that there was a gap between the pervasiveness of pain questionnaires as diagnostic tools in the global north and their relatively recent and uneven arrival in Indian pain practice.

Misgivings about copyright aside, a more fundamental concern exercised these participants against global pain diagnostic questionnaires. The point of friction they identified in the translation of such instruments formulated elsewhere was that the instruments were not attuned to the spiritual orientation of Indian patients. At first, I was not surprised by this insistence on the importance of spirituality in Indian emotional life. Through the British colonial period, the region was associated with an otherworldly ascetic ethic. Its inhabitants were imagined by Europeans as predisposed to a transcendental negation of this-worldly sensations and experiences, and death and pain were understood as exemplary of detachment and equanimity.[23] Anthropologists and historians working in the region have demonstrated how this characterization of the subcontinent lent itself to the colonial project. If native subjects were understood to be more concerned with otherworldly matters, then it was the task of the colonizer to provide them with a grounded political orientation—that is, the colonial government.[24] Similarly, contemporary American medical ethics textbooks, journals, and monographs look to India to teach the "West" to be more accepting of death and to resist Euro-American trends toward overmedicalization.[25] Thus, it seemed plausible to me that contemporary Indian research would echo these past constructions of pain. The conference evidenced many such reverberations. In a panel on palliative care ethics, the backgrounds of several slide-shows were composed of faded-out tableaux of Hindu gods and goddesses. Ethical guidelines about "dying well" from Hindu scriptural texts were laid over these tableaux, intended to urge doctors to pay attention to particularly Indian spiritual needs. Later, at a training session on how to communicate a terminal prognosis, participants were urged to look for signs of religious orientations and to temper their communication using the vocabularies of resilience and forbearance found in "Hindu" religious belief.

To take a longer view, research into the relation between ascetic transcendence and culturally "Indian" practices at AIIMS is as old as the institute itself. In 1952, a French cardiologist, Therese Brosse, traveled to Delhi to conduct experiments on yogis to explore their ability to control their heart and respiration. She had already visited in 1936 on a French medical mission and had tested the famous yogi Tirumalai Krishnamacharya, with positive results for her claim.[26] During her 1952 visit, she could not conduct her experiments because an electroencephalograph that she had sought to import from America did not arrive in time. The machine finally arrived in 1957 and was installed at AIIMS. In 1961, a team of three researchers—from UCLA, the University of Michigan, and AIIMS—sought to confirm Brosse's finding, even retesting her original subject.[27] Their conclusions prevaricated on Brosse's claim. They suggested that the machine Brosse had used was not sensitive enough to record what they found: that some of the yogis could significantly slow their hearts, but none could stop it. Another example of research with the electroencephalograph at the institute was conducted on Shri Ramanand Yogi, who was studied in an airtight sealed box for ten hours (figure 3.5).[28] The study concluded that by controlling basic involuntary biological mechanisms, the yogi could significantly reduce his oxygen intake and carbon dioxide output.

As William Broad describes it, experiments such as these sought to move asceticism from a science of the spectacular and mystical to one that was measurable, biological, and observable.[29] Drawing on Projit Mukharji's analysis of Ayurveda in a different time period, the reconceptualization of asceticism might be described as a shift from a pataphysics to metaphysics: from a science of the singular, the unrepeatable, and the inexplicable, to a science of explicability and representability.[30] In other words, if pataphysics acknowledged limits of generalizability and understanding, the new mod-

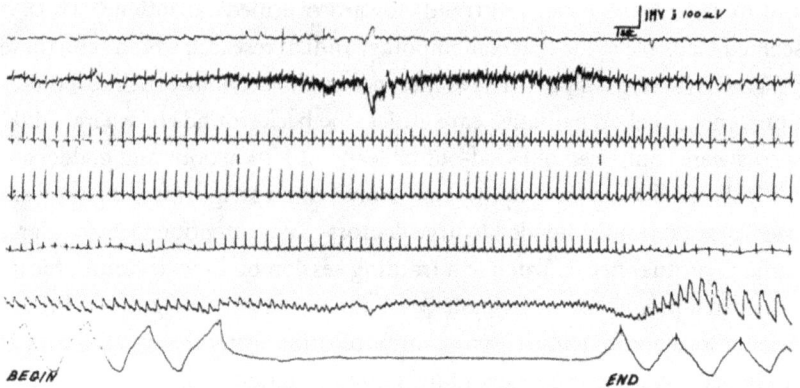

FIGURE 3.5 EEG report from an AIIMS study on Shri Ramanand Yogi's ability to voluntarily "stop" his metabolism and respiration. From B. K. Anand, G. S. Chinna, and B. Singh, "Studies on Shri Ramanand Yogi during His Stay in an Air-Tight Box," *Indian Journal of Medical Research* 49, no. 1 (1961): 88.

ern postcolonial metaphysics was amenable to representations in machines such as the electroencephalograph. This early work at AIIMS was crucial in opening the domain of the mystical and spiritual to measurable biomedical research. The collaborator on the Brosse confirmation research—Dr. Bal K. Anand—would continue research on yogic practices over the next two decades at AIIMS. By 1969, Dr. Anand's collaborator, Dr. Chinna, claimed that more than five hundred yogis had been tested in the first two decades of the institute, and that the team at AIIMS were close to putting yoga on a "rational basis."[31] Even as studies such as these continued through the postcolonial decades, the turn of the twenty-first century saw an exponential increase in the scale of such research. Whereas somewhere between 10 and 30 studies were published in five-year periods from 1967 to 2003, the number tripled to 76 for the period between 2004 and 2008, and then tripled again to 243 between 2009 and 2013.[32] It was also around the turn of the century that I found the relation between spirituality and cancer pain emerging as a biomedical research concern in India.

One of the first articulations of cancer pain as a problematic appeared in 1998, in a clinical psychology study that sought to understand culture as a factor in how patients dealt with terminal cancer diagnoses (figure 3.6).[33] This early study set a precedent for foregrounding spirituality and a theory of karma as strongly determining a patient's ability to cope with cancer. Positing that metaphysical beliefs strongly influenced psychological well-being,

Table 2

Correlations of Causal Beliefs with Perceived Controllability and
Measures of Psychological Recovery (N = 132)

Causal Beliefs	Perceived Controllability	Perceived Recovery (Measure 1)	Reactions to Crisis (Measure 2)	Psychological Recovery (Measures 1 + 2)
Fate	−.22*	.07	−.06	−.03
God's Will	−.22*	.20*	.11	.15
Karmaphala	−.12	−.04	−.12	−.10
Own Carelessness	.04	−.14	−.08	−.10
Bodily Weakness	−.04	−.16	−.25**	−.24**
Mental Stress	−.05	−.30**	−.36**	−.36**
Family Circumstances	−.03	−.26**	−.31**	−.31**
Other's Negligence	.23**	−.12	−.13	−.14

Notes: *p < .05.   **p < .01.

FIGURE 3.6 Table from a study that measured the relation between beliefs about illness and psychological recovery. From Neena Kohli and Ajit K. Dalal, "Culture as a Factor in Causal Understanding of Illness: A Study of Cancer Patients," *Psychology and Developing Societies* 10, no. 2 (1998): 123.

the authors concluded that patients who attributed illness to God's will and karma (rather than physical etiology) were better equipped to deal with cancer-related psychiatric distress. A study published two years later developed this hypothesis by studying the correlation between spiritual belief and recovery across a range of life-threatening diagnoses, including tuberculosis, heart disease, and cancer (figure 3.7).[34] In this second study, the results confounded researchers. It appeared that in some diseases, a Hindu attribution of disease to a transcendent religious will helped in coping and recovery, while in others it hindered psychological well-being. These conflicting results pushed subsequent researchers in opposite directions. Some researchers wondered whether the effect of religious beliefs was too varied for statistical quantification; others hoped that they could resolve these anomalies through an accounting for a broader range of variables. As transcendent Indian spirituality became a central theme, it led to practical suggestions for therapeutic management. Several studies suggested that "spirituality" did indeed offer a powerful coping mechanism and that Indian practitioners should incorporate it into therapy.[35] Others suggested that research questionnaires needed to be modified to account for the role of Indian spirituality in psychiatric well-being.[36] At present, one of the leading researchers on this theme

Table 4

Correlation of Health Beliefs with Psychological Recovery/ Adjustment Measures

	TB	MI	Cancer	Orthopaedic Temp	Perm
n =	70	70	114	20	21
Causal Beliefs					
Own Carelessness	.22	.30**	−.10	.30	.01
Other's Carelessness	−.24**	.01	−.14	.11	.25
Family Conditions	.26**	.02	−.31***	−.06	−.14
Fate/Chance	−.15	–	−.03	–	–
God's will	−.09	−.37***	.15	−.05	.29
Karma	−.06	−.19	−.10	.39*	.29
Recovery Beliefs					
Self	.05	.24*	.28***	–	
Family	−.03	−.06	.16	–	
Money	.08	–	–	–	
Fate/chance	−.28**	–	.11	–	
God	−.29**	.29**	.09	–	
Karma	.18	.29**	.02	–	
Doctor	−.12	−.18	.00	–	
Control Beliefs					
Self	.40***	.21	.04		
Disease	.18	.33**	.29**		

Notes: *p<.10, **p<.05, ***p<.01.
Temp = Temporary; Perm = Permanent.

FIGURE 3.7 Table from a study that measured the relation between beliefs about illness and psychological adjustment across different illness groups. From Ajit K. Dalal, "Living with a Chronic Disease: Healing and Psychological Adjustment in Indian Society," *Psychology and Developing Societies* 12, no. 1 (2000): 76.

is Dr. Santosh Chaturvedi, professor of psychiatry at the National Institute of Mental Health and Neurosciences. One of India's leading psychiatrists, he has published a range of clinical studies suggesting that particular forms of spiritual satisfaction correlate with "Indian" psychiatric well-being.[37] The broader implication of his work and the work of others on the theme was that if the "materialistic West" understood happiness materially and functionally, spiritual welfare might be an important dimension of well-being in India.

In 2016, Dr. Chaturvedi and a team of authors including Dr. Nigam (as well as researchers from the United States and Europe) collaborated on a research project at AIIMS to produce a spiritual questionnaire for Indian cancer patients.[38] This study was the most sophisticated attempt yet to coalesce the decades of interest in spirituality and pain into a concrete diagnostic tool. Much like my collaborative attempt to produce an appropriate "psychosocial" questionnaire, it aimed to assess the "spiritual" dimension of cancer pain. In consonance with the literature they drew upon, the researchers found a connection between spirituality and transcendence, understanding spiritual belief to be a belief in a power, force, or entity that transcended human life. Operationalizing this conception of spirituality, they set out to validate their initial questionnaire, enlisting three hundred patients at AIIMS as research subjects. Based on this questionnaire, this prospective study argued that most Indian cancer patients derived support from their relationship with the divine. The researchers also reported that older patients were more likely to bear the burden of an "existential blame"—attributing their disease to their own bad karma, sin, or wrongdoing. As for a correlation between spirituality and the intensity of pain, the study found that higher degrees of pain correlated with patients questioning their religious views and their belief in God. At the same time, the study recognized that earlier work had not found clear correlations between spirituality and the intensity of pain, and that the phenomenon of "spirituality" might be too complex to serve up clear, unambiguous correlations with pain scores. A year later, a follow-up study that included the original authors sought to find out the most common signs of spiritual distress from the same data, and to explore gender differences in these results. In this follow-up, the authors conceded that patients might exaggerate their belief in God in such interviews, conforming to wider Indian societal expectations to express religiosity. Yet, the authors contended, this did not invalidate what they believed to be the patients' genuine longing for spiritual peace and divine support.

The emphasis on spiritual transcendence in studies such as these bears some traces of historical constructions of Indian spirituality. It is impossible to disentangle two centuries of European and native interest in ascetic resilience from the contemporary biomedical discourse about a particularly "Indian" capacity to invoke spirituality as a response to cancer pain. Yet, these long historical imprints are, at best, just traces; it is difficult to draw direct lines of influence from a colonial past to the contemporary future. The more proximate and explicit referents of such research are "new religious movements" that have become immensely popular among the Indian middle classes. Gurus of such movements seductively blend the languages of self-help, business-speak, and science, claiming to reinvent "old" traditions for the challenges of the contemporary world. Tulasi Srinivas describes the leaders of these movements as "hyper-gurus" who can build a global coalition of devotees and transnational infrastructures of support.[39] Further, Joanne Waghorne pinpoints their special popularity among technological professionals in global Asian cities, who are drawn to their guru's seamless mixing of business, scientific, and putatively "Hindu" vocabularies.[40] While working at AIIMS, I saw how in an interdepartmental project between the cancer institute and the department of neurology, one such new religious movement found its way into the research on cancer pain. This project sought to determine the effect of yogic practices on easing cancer-related distress. The practices identified for testing were Sudarshan Kriya, a set of exercises codified by the influential guru Sri Sri Ravi Shankar as the core component of the Art of Living. The goals of the Art of Living movement are seductively simple and nondoctrinal—to relieve stress, resolve conflict, and improve health. According to the movement's own estimate, it has more than 350 million followers worldwide. Ravi Shankar began his career working with Maharishi Mahesh Yogi in Switzerland, returning to India in 1981 to start the movement in Bangalore. The growth of the movement coincided with the explosion of IT firms in the city; middle-class entrepreneurs and businesses would become its chief followers. Nandini Gooptu argues that the movement articulates well with a middle-class politics of personal growth and responsibility; for example, she quotes Ravi Shankar as stating that those who demand rights from the state are weak.[41]

Ravi Shankar's influence has been significant at AIIMS, where some doctors at the cancer institute sign off research papers acknowledging his inspirational teaching. Much like the engineers described by Waghorne, the predominantly middle-class doctors at the cancer hospital were particularly open to his adept blending of scientific, religious, and self-help vocabularies. In part, his influence was routed through Dr. Panikkar, who joined AIIMS in 1975. She became the head of medical oncology in 1986, then rose to the highest position in the cancer institute as its chief director in 1992, a post she held until 2008. Having published more than a hundred research papers, she is one of the most prolific authors at the hospital. Through her time at AIIMS, Dr. Panikkar has been a strong proponent of the Art of Living movement. During her time as department head, she organized several international workshops and conferences on the benefits of Kriya for cancer patients, bringing in psychiatrists and oncologists from all over the world. She also worked alongside the Department of Physiology to set up a yoga space called the Integral Health Clinic. Although she was no longer the chief at the cancer hospital when I conducted my fieldwork, I was able to sit in on a presentation she conducted for the staff on the benefits of Kriya. The talk began with an informal poll that asked, "Are you happy with your life?" When most members of the audience halfheartedly raised their hands, her reveal was that this poll was contrary to studies that show a high prevalence of depression and anxiety in India. She went on to talk about the mind-body connection and about neuropeptides as the "molecules of emotion." This then led to her describing a perfect match between a map of chakras and of neuropeptides arranged along the spine. Having thus laid the ground for a relation between mind, body, and indigenous systems of knowledge, she introduced the Art of Living movement. Aware of her biomedical audience, she stressed the relation between Kriya, peptides, the frontal cortex, and endorphins. To demonstrate her point, she displayed electroencephalography (EEG) charts that showed a marked difference between those who practiced Kriya and those who did not. Her broader claim was that practicing Kriya increased "natural killer cells" and the body's "antioxidant defense," slowing down cancer progression. The presentation ended with a quote from Sri Sri Ravi Shankar: "The systematic understanding of reality is called science and systematic understanding of one who is understanding is called spirituality."

In consonance with this blending of medicine and Art of Living, a series of recent clinical trials at the cancer hospital have sought to show the positive effects of Kriya and other forms of yoga on immune function, tobacco addictions, antioxidant status, and blood lactose levels. In 2004, Dr. Panikkar assisted an EEG-based study conducted on two groups of policemen. After six months, the experimental group was found to exhibit far lower levels of stress than the control group. A major pilot study between the cancer hospital and the Department of Biochemistry at AIIMS in 2008 identified positive effects of Kriya at the level of gene expression. During my fieldwork, I was able to follow a project that was the newest iteration of the theme of cancer and yogic practice. The team of doctors I worked with at AIIMS included a resident physiotherapist intern, Shilpa. A young woman in her twenties, Shilpa was placed in charge of a clinical research project to study the effects of yogic practice on cancer patients. The study was undertaken and funded in collaboration with the Ministry of Ayurveda, Yoga and Naturopathy, Unani, Siddha and Homoeopathy (AYUSH), a government body set up in 1995 under the National Ministry of Health and Family Welfare to encourage research into alternative health systems. The researchers at the cancer hospital focused on two forms of yogic practice: Kriya and Pranayama (exercises focused on the breath). This 2012 study sought to find out the influence of the combined practices on pain and stress among advanced-stage breast cancer patients. Shilpa would recruit eligible patients from the outpatient and inpatient clinics of the institute and then train them for in-dividual practice. This preliminary training took place over eighteen hours, spanning three days. Acknowledging the inability of poorer patients to re-peatedly make their way to AIIMS, Shilpa taught them basic techniques they could practice at home. The team also developed a simple version of a self-monitoring chart that patients would be responsible for over two to three months. At the end of this period, they would report to the institute for tests, including the measurement of their serotonin levels (a neurotransmitter as-sociated with feelings of well-being and happiness).

Shilpa's task was not an easy one. Human subjects research on vulnerable cancer patients has had a difficult history in India, as in many other parts of the world. For example, in 1997, the *British Medical Journal* threatened to blacklist all research published by biomedical researchers in India. This was after it was revealed that the Indian Council for Medical Research had sanctioned cervical cancer research that did not inform 1,100 patients about the existence of precancerous lesions, leading to 62 of these women devel-oping cancer. While AIIMS was later absolved of participation in this trial, the cloud never lifted from its inclusion in the accusation.[42] As rumors of clinical research malpractice abound, lower-income patients justifiably feel anxious about becoming unwitting research subjects in trials they do not fully understand, and might never benefit from.[43] To ensure the compliance of advanced-stage patients, Shilpa had to follow up with nearly every one of her recruits, grapple with high dropout rates, and fight for the resource-constrained testing facilities at the biochemistry department. She managed to enroll 147 patients in the trial and, miraculously, was able to convince them to come back for three-day workshops when large enough groups had been assembled.[44]

Conducting the trial involved Shilpa spending long hours at work well beyond the normal clinic schedule. She was already vital to the pain and palliative care team, which called on her to help negotiate the large influx of patients in the outpatient wards. The clinical trial made a heavy demand on the time of both the patients and the staff of the cancer institute. Yet, as its current flagship research project, conducting the trial was a priority that neither its administrators nor its participants could ignore. When the study was concluded, its authors reported that 78 percent of the interven-tion group regularly practiced what they were taught in the workshop.[45] The authors admitted that it had been difficult to determine whether subjects were able to follow the strict practice schedule when they were at home. Fi-nally, the authors concluded that they had found a statistically significant difference between the cortisol levels of those who had received standard biomedical treatment and those who received the standard treatment supplemented with Kriya and Pranayama. Celebrating the positive result, the authors suggested that this kind of therapeutic intervention was wonderful, since it could be universally applied: yoga could be "uniformly followed across the countries, irrespective of cast [sic] creed." Bolstered by two decades of such research across the cancer institute as well as at other departments at AIIMS, a new Center for Integrative Medicine and Research was inaugurated in the hospital in 2016. The four-thousand-square-foot facility houses a massive yoga studio and an Ayurveda and naturopathy center. In inaugurating the facility, the Indian health minister J. P. Nadda identified its cost-effectiveness benefits for the poor and stated that it was another step in the government's goal of continuing to shift focus away from treatment and toward well-being and prevention.[46] Because noncommunicable diseases were primarily caused by lifestyles, he added, they could be "easily cured by practicing yoga," even in "malignant" cases.[47] As I discussed in the introduction, the context of Nadda's statements is a long shift in government policy away from treatment and toward behavioral modification. They reveal the continuing implications of framing noncommunicable diseases as "lifestyle" problems. In this instance, a proposed "Eastern" practice is operationalized to treat cancer, a disease associated with "Western" lifestyles.

In tracking this orientation in biomedical research on cancer pain in India, and particularly at AIIMS, I thus found sincere efforts to conceptualize cancer pain as more than its physical etiologies and biological damage. Through measurable and evidence-based research, palliative cancer care researchers and physicians sought to expand the definition of pain to encapsulate further dimensions and etiologies, variously understood—the "social," "psychological," and "spiritual." At the same time, in enacting this desire to expand the etiological boundaries of cancer pain, they often took recourse to old and new vocabularies of resilience and transcendence. The "psychosocial" that came into being was a manifestation of these contextual conjunctures, diffusing pain through the capacities of the putative "Indian" mind.

To my mind, even as this research promises novel therapeutic approaches to dealing with the distress of cancer patients, it frames the extrabiological in ways that might need some rethinking. Its explicit focus on "transcendence" reveals in sharp relief the absence of research on the more this-worldly socioeconomic forms of affliction. To think of this in another way, palliative care research frames existential concerns (the waxing and waning of faith, of divine support, of the cause and blame for misfortune) as separate and distinct from the difficulties of everyday life. This, despite Dr. Nigam's perceptive claim in one published piece that poverty was perhaps the most crucial factor contributing to the suffering of Indian cancer patients. My intention here is not to call into question the growing interest in the spiritual dimensions of pain. More recent work (particularly the collaborative research at AIIMS that involves health care researchers across the United States and Europe) has taken seriously the multidimensionality of what a concept like spirituality might mean and acknowledged the difficulty in finding correspondences between its many dimensions and intensities. However, I suggest that thickening this research, framing the "spiritual" as growing out of everyday life and not emerging as above and apart from it, will reveal new directions for understanding the existential dimensions of cancer pain. As I have described in prior chapters, feelings of anger, blame, hope, and helplessness are rooted in the everyday worlds in which cancer appears, and not primarily dependent on religious and cultural beliefs that stand apart from social life. If palliative cancer care research aims to identify the transcendental and the otherworldly as sites of both distress and support, my aim here is to continue to put the otherworldly in conversation with more immanent concerns.

Acknowledging Limits

In my first few days of working at this palliative care unit, I encountered Hardeep Singh, a patient whose name I had heard mentioned in several conversations. He was the stuff of lore among pain professionals in Delhi. In conferences, talks, and meetings, discussions of his case would bring together practitioners who might never have met before. Hardeep was a sixty-four-year-old man who first came to the hospital in 2001 with a rare, fast-growing malignant mesenchymal tumor lodged in the bones of his right leg. Following the treatment protocol for this cancer, his leg was amputated above the knee. Hardeep returned to the hospital after ten days, showing telltale signs of phantom limb pain. He had already been prescribed oral morphine, and then Dr. Nigam increased the dosage. This was the first of many visits that continued until the time of my research. He would present with only partial pain relief, sometimes resulting in a further escalation of his morphine dosage. At other times, he would be admitted to the inpatient unit for more serious interventions. His relationship with Dr. Nigam had grown over this time. She had tried every available therapeutic option, delving deep into the biomedical literature on phantom limb pain. These had included intravenous opioids, ketamine, electrical nerve stimulations, and a range of semi-invasive surgeries placing spinal cord stimulators, neuromodulators, and nerve blocks within his body. Hardeep's pain resisted each of these interventions. Through Dr. Nigam, Hardeep availed himself of therapies as advanced as any offered by the best pain clinics anywhere in the world. Yet, the only thing that provided him any measure of relief was oral morphine. And so, over the next decade, Dr. Nigam slowly raised his dose. By the time I met Hardeep, he was prescribed more than 1,200 mg of morphine a day, along with other pain-relieving medications.

Given his decade-long pain biography, only Dr. Nigam and a few other veteran oncologists had been at the cancer hospital as long as Hardeep. New junior residents often worried about the possibility of his addiction to his high morphine dosage and the "truth" of his mysterious pain. One junior resident went as far as to doubt even the existence of a baseline pain and attributed all Hardeep's actions to drug-seeking behavior, asking, "We've titrated his dose for over ten years, we've tried every block, every experimental procedure, nothing has worked. His pain is not physical. Should we not try psychiatric de-addiction therapies?" This was a familiar question for Dr. Nigam, one that many cohorts of residents had asked her before. As she had with his predecessors, she urged this new resident to think beyond the "easy" answer of addiction: "It is difficult to call him an addict. Yes, we should try it [de-addiction], and I will recommend an appointment with a psychiatrist. But pay attention to how he talks about his pain, how he always describes it in the same way, and how its intensity matches the dose. They are all classic symptoms of phantom limb. Go do your research, see if there are newer pain therapies we could try." In fact, they had already sent Hardeep to the hospital's de-addiction specialists to guard against this line of questioning. I never met the psychiatrist, but I was told that Hardeep had been cleared of the charge of "drug-seeking behavior."

Dr. Nigam's haste to clear Hardeep of the charge of addiction was crucial to maintaining their long-standing therapeutic relationship. As Helena Hansen and Mary Skinner have shown in their work on analgesic politics in the United States, long histories of politically stratified assumptions about patients and their psychiatric states lie behind the marketing and prescription of opioid painkillers.[48] Medical morphine is heavily controlled by the Indian state. In 1985, the Narcotics Drugs and Psychotropic Substances Act criminalized morphine, with a ten-year minimum mandatory sentence for prescription-related abuse. It also put in place bureaucratic hurdles for hospitals and pharmacies seeking to stock the drug. Thus, while the act might have aimed to curtail addiction, palliative care specialists like Dr. Nigam argue that one consequence of its implementation has been the virtual disappearance of morphine from institutional medical practice in India. It took five years for the cancer care NGO that I describe in chapters 4 and 5 to negotiate a license to prescribe the drug to its terminally ill patients. At the same time, India remained the largest licit producer of raw opium in the world market, accounting for nearly 90 percent of global production. In 1998, two physicians filed a public interest litigation suit in the Delhi High Court, demanding the drug for cancer patients. Their mother had died of the disease a year earlier, and despite their connections with the pharmaceutical industry, they claimed they had been unable to procure any licit morphine. Their litigation led to the relaxation of licensing rules in eight out of India's twenty-nine states, including Delhi. Cansupport and Dr. Nigam's lobbying of the Delhi Drug Control Department had particularly eased restrictions in the region in 2007. Yet, through the course of my fieldwork in Delhi in 2011–2012, I found that doctors (apart for those at AIIMS) would often prescribe acetaminophen (Tylenol) or ibuprofen (Advil) for many instances of cancer pain.

However, most doctors campaigning for the availability of morphine—including Dr. Nigam—contend that the Narcotics Act did far more damage than just restrict legal sales. They suggest that it produced a climate of fear among pharmacists and doctors, even in places like Delhi that have seen the most legal reform. I encountered this fear of prescription when I sat in on one of Dr. Nigam's many training sessions in hospitals across the city. I sat in the audience as Dr. Nigam cited several studies that showed the relative absence of opioid addiction among terminally ill cancer patients. She went further to claim there was not a single documented case of opioid addiction among the cancer patients she had treated at AIIMS. While I was unfamiliar with the research she cited, I wondered at the strong concern about addiction among terminally ill patients who had little time to live in the first place. I was sitting in the audience with a general physician I had struck up a conversation with, and I asked him what he thought. He responded that he respected Dr. Nigam's expertise and thought she perhaps was right about morphine being the most effective therapy. But, he continued, the patients he saw would not understand the strict rules about how, when, and how much of it to take. He had enough on his hands, without the added hassle of dealing with a police case, if something were to go wrong. Throughout my fieldwork, I found echoes of his assumptions among middle-and upper-class doctors about poorer patients' propensity toward addiction and illicit use.

To be clear, this is not to say that opioid abuse is not a problem in India and that the doctors' assumptions of a prevalence of addiction were necessarily wrong.[49] However, my aim here is not to evaluate the claims of morphine addiction in Delhi; rather, I am interested in how claims about the absence or presence of addiction guided palliative cancer care. In this regard, the difficulty of procuring licit morphine was the most cited concern expressed by the physicians I worked with. They published on, lectured on, and campaigned for public recognition that cancer patients did not abuse prescription analgesics, and they simultaneously produced and drew upon the discourse of an epidemic of untreated cancer pain. A statistic that recurred in their claims was that only 0.4 percent of cancer patients in India who needed morphine had licit access to the drug.[50] It is within this discursive context of an epidemic of cancer pain that Dr. Nigam sought to treat and rehabilitate Hardeep. Her aversion toward the quick label of addiction was a careful and strategic act, designed to keep at bay accusations of abuse and unregulated drug use. To call Hardeep an addict would place him in de-addiction interventions and could remove him from Dr. Nigam's direct care. In the severely controlled world of opiate regulation in India, she believed it could also lead to his decisive, long-term severance from future licit prescription. Further, cases such as these would compromise her continuing efforts to lobby the Delhi government and would dilute her argument that there had not been a documented case of opioid addiction among her cancer patients.

Toward the end of my time at AIIMS, Dr. Nigam threw a party at her home for past and current residents of the pain clinic. The conversation at the party drifted to Hardeep's condition, with one of the older residents narrating the following story. When the resident had joined the clinic, he had asked Hardeep in a tone of incredulity about his lack of relief from his high morphine dosage. He had even asked Hardeep if he had tried counseling and meditation. Hardeep had shot back, "You're new here, aren't you?" The memory of this quip evoked laughter all around. The conversation turned then to the "truth" of Hardeep's condition. A senior resident said elliptically, "With pain, you never know." Most nodded in agreement. Thus, while residents would continue to try every possible therapeutic option, Hardeep's phantom pain would meanwhile serve as a disciplinary reminder of the limits of what the pain specialists could do. While newer residents responded to Hardeep with suspicion, older residents allowed the recalcitrance of Hardeep's pain to teach them lessons in humility. Both shared an openness to the idea that Hardeep's pain was "real," and that, in any case, if morphine helped ease his complaints, then so be it.

This theme of Hardeep's recalcitrant pain as a point of learning continued when I visited him in his home with Cansupport. After a treacherous car ride through the narrow by-lanes of a West Delhi housing community, we abandoned our car some distance from Hardeep's house. In collaboration with Dr. Nigam, the Cansupport team I was visiting him with had recently tried the well-known mirror box therapy devised by the Indian American neuroscientist V. Ramachandran. The mirror box is designed to trick the mind into seeing the amputated limb in a reflection of the existing physical limb. The phantom limb is thus made to appear real, allowing the patient to work through the virtual pain through physical exercises. The mirror box exercise perfectly illustrates the neuroscientific consensus on locating conditions of pain primarily in the brain. That is, if pain exists only as a virtual neuronal image, the malleability of the brain can be engaged by tricking it into believing a virtual limb exists, and then training it to release the limb's phantom pain. In Hardeep's case, however, the therapy had met with repeated failure. Instead, Hardeep continued to describe his pain through his own metaphors. The metaphors he drew upon were those that were most real to him from before his illness, when he had worked as a furniture maker. Pointing to his real limb, he described the pain in his absent limb as being like the hammering of nails and the cutting of a saw. Most of our visits consisted of the home-care team patiently listening to Hardeep narrate the events of his week, followed sometimes by adjustments to his morphine dosage that were punctuated by his descriptions of his recalcitrant pain. Sometime later, I visited Hardeep with a counselor who was new to the profession. This counselor tried to distract Hardeep with conversation about his family and his grandchildren, urging him to think of the time that had passed since his amputation and of the comfort that his familial life must provide. In response, all he received was Hardeep's famous condescension. The more experienced doctor who had been collaborating with Dr. Nigam for several years winced at the counselor's intervention. Later, she would privately tell me that perhaps this failure was for the best; it was a way for the counselor to learn the limits of what they could do.

Phantom limb pain is not the only type of cancer-related pain, nor is it even necessarily the most common. Like most kinds of cancer pain, it is related to the type of cancer, its correspondent damage, the nature of treatments, and the stage of the cancer's progression. I focus on it here primarily because of the particular problem it raises for pain physicians. As a kind of pain, it is without a specifiable location. It epitomizes the inherent and much-discussed difficulty of empathizing with pain: to relate to the pain of another is often to relate to something invisible, to take as fact a feeling one does not feel or cannot even see.[51] The repetitive mantra of palliative care—of seeing through the patient's eyes—was then both a recognition of this problem of empathy and a wager that empathy in such conditions of doubt was still possible. To treat Hardeep's pain, the pain physicians had to take him at his word, moving past the cloud of his possible addiction. Dr. Nigam's pedagogical impulse was to introduce this problem of recognition and to communicate the necessity of staking their pain practice on trust. To see through the patient's eyes was *not* to directly feel the experience of the patient. Rather, it was to take the pain as real, attuned to the possibility of its intractability.

This orientation at AIIMS becomes clearer when put in relief against other biomedical approaches to phantom limb pain. In almost every work of contemporary pain science, a paper coauthored in 1965 by the neuroscientist Patrick Wall and the psychologist Ronald Melzack is cited as having laid the foundations for pain research.[52] As Melzack has written since, in that paper they sought to correct a three-century-old biological model of pain therapeutics inherited from Descartes. For Melzack and Wall, prior pain theories presented an all-too-simple relationship between bodily damage and the nature and extent of pain as the body's response. They argued that this led to the devaluation of the psychological etiologies of chronic pain, since chronic patients often could not present signs of obvious organic damage. Instead, the "gate-control theory" proposed by Melzack and Wall emphasized the central nervous system and the brain as constituting an active system that filters and modulates sensory stimuli. Thus, the "psychological" factors of chronic pain (previously devalued as not real, since they had no biological basis) could now be understood as dynamically modulating the perception of pain. Through an appeal to the malleability of the central nervous system, pain physicians learned to understand psychological experience as central to pain. Because pain experience was no longer equated with physical damage, psychological factors such as past experience became legitimate therapeutic concerns.

However, in 1990, Melzack revised his earlier position and proposed a new refined hypothesis: the "neuromatrix" theory of pain.[53] The explanatory power of the neuromatrix theory lay in its claim of having solved the problem of phantom limb pain. The condition had resisted the gate-control theory, which still rested on the presence of some form of physical damage or sensory input. The new theory proposed that a matrix of neurons produces characteristic nerve impulse patterns for the body and its somatosensory apparatus. The neuromatrix theory purported to explain not only how physiological damage produced unanticipated patterns of dispersed pain (often found in cancer pain) but also, and more ambitiously, how pain could exist in the absence of any sensory input at all (such as with phantom limb pain). Thus, as Melzack writes, "Phantoms become comprehensible once we recognize the brain generates the experience of the body."[54] It is only by considering this neuronal theory of pain that the mirror box intervention to relieve phantom limb pain makes sense. If phantom pain can be found and localized in the brain, it can be alleviated by briefly tricking the brain into believing that the absent limb—evidenced by the mirror—is not absent after all.

The pain physicians at AIIMS were both part of this biomedical tradition and departed from it. In one study, Dr. Nigam described phantom pain thus: "The mechanisms for phantom phenomenon are complex and involve various elements in the somatic pain generators, peripheral nervous system, spinal cord, and brain." Following the broader biomedical consensus on research into phantom limb pain, she too located it biologically—dispersing it across parts of the body—especially in the nervous system and the brain. Following from this, she attempted several interventionist pain therapies. At the same time, she remained open to the possibility of the ongoing intractability of Hardeep's pain, even if it could not be precisely located in biological damage. Taking Hardeep as a paradigmatic case, she taught newer specialists to attend to pain while remaining attuned to the possibility of therapeutic failure. At the margins of the heroic interventions of curative oncology, these physicians worked within and through the uncertainties and long temporality of pain that could not easily be localized and removed. Allowing Hardeep's phantom limb pain to rest somewhere between the possibility of addiction and truth, Dr. Nigam took this pain as a lesson about limits. The virtual excess of phantom limb pain—its unclear etiologies and resistance to imaging and treatment—was the point at which she turned her spade.

A Shared Death

At the palliative care ward, this pedagogy of limits was confined not only to pain but also to the ever-present possibility of death. If witnessing intractable pain taught practitioners to acknowledge the limits of their intervention and to acknowledge and trust the voice of the patient, the reminders of mortality in a cancer ward demanded similar efforts at recognition and empathy. But, as I describe here, if phantom limb pain resisted easy translation from patient to physician, the fact of mortality was something that physicians could claim to share.

At the time of my fieldwork, Dr. Arjun was the most senior resident in the cancer pain and palliative care unit at AIIMS. Many other residents echoed the narrative of his turn to palliative care. Like Dr. Abha, his first serious introduction to palliative care and chronic cancer pain was not through his training as an anesthesiologist but under Dr. Nigam's tutelage at AIIMS. While many of his friends had left for the lucrative prospects of the United States after medical school, he had instead joined AIIMS. Then, three years ago (he cited the exact date as if it to underline its significance), his chest X-ray had showed the possibility of tumorous growth. He explained his reaction to this discovery in the following way:

> I can't explain to you what that did to me. I spent the entire day thinking, knowing, I was going to die a painful death within the next six months, that's the prognosis with that kind of carcinoma. I didn't tell my wife or my parents. The next day I had a CT scan, where I reacted badly to the dye. Anyway, it turned out to be nonmalignant, and not even a cancer-related growth. I could only tell my wife after finding out that it wasn't malignant, and she's also a doctor! I couldn't tell my parents over the phone, I had to wait to physically see them. Every time I look at a patient, and I tend to lose my temper sometimes, but as soon as I think of this, I can't help but see the world *through their eyes* [italics added]. Trust me when I say this, anyone can get cancer, anyone. I don't drink, I don't smoke, but it nearly happened to me. Every time I have to get an X-ray now— there's a 20 percent chance of recurrence, so I have to get an X-ray every year—I have to really work up the courage to go.

A few weeks later, Dr. Arjun walked into the residents' office looking visibly distraught. He sat down at the computer next to me, clicking distractedly. Before long, unable to maintain his usual studied reserve, he sought a conversation. "I'm glad you're here, I don't really want to be alone right now." A patient the residents had all been close to, Kamini, was nearing the end of her life. Kamini was the wife of a member of the department's cleaning staff, twenty-nine years old and the mother of a four-month-old child. She had been battling the quick progression of her disease for the last year.

In that year, Dr. Arjun and Dr. Nigam had been particularly attentive to her care, in part because they were the ones closest to her husband. In the past few days, Kamini's condition had quickly deteriorated. While talking, Dr. Arjun added, "You've never been married. You can't know what this feels like." I remembered that his own daughter was just a few months older than the patient's child. Gathering himself, he returned to the inpatient ward where Kamini was admitted. A few minutes later, he returned and said, fighting through his tears, "She just passed." A little while later, Dr. Mohit—another senior resident—walked into the office. He had sensed that Dr. Arjun needed consolation. Over the next hour, they talked about how it was not the fact of death that scared patients but the desolation of the family members they left behind. Dr. Arjun and Dr. Mohit filled out the death certificate and paused over whether it was a "natural" or "unnatural" death, mulling over whether those categories really meant anything. There was some indecision about whether the cause of death was to be attributed to coronary failure, to the advanced progression of the malignancy, or to both. Dr. Mohit presented a stoic demeanor, saying, "I have got used to all this." Moments later, however, he turned to me to rhetorically ask, "How can anyone believe in God at a time like this?"

After a while, Dr. Mohit left the room to attend to the business of the inpatient ward. It was only then that Dr. Arjun told me that Dr. Mohit's father was in critical care at that moment, having struggled with multiple myeloma (a cancer of the plasma cells) for almost ten years. Dr. Mohit had first come to AIIMS not as a doctor but as a son accompanying his elderly father, queuing at the same outpatient lines he now administered. A few days later, I would find out that over the past ten years, his father had been in and out of critical care, and with each admission attending oncologists had told Dr. Mohit to give up and prepare for the end. Dr. Arjun said, quietly and with admiration, "He has single-handedly brought his father back to life, not once, but four times." He then described how his own cancer scare had changed his outlook on his work: "I used to have a bad temper before the diagnosis, and like many other oncologists here, I could not help but shout at patients when I thought they did not understand what I was saying. You know, we Indian doctors have a bad reputation for being angry. But after that incident, I have learned to become more of a palliative specialist. I try to wonder what it must feel like for them. You know, cancer is a disease that anyone can get. *There's no difference between them and me* [italics added]." When Dr. Mohit came back in, they talked first about a friend's wife who had been diagnosed with cervical cancer a few months after marriage. I asked both doctors about how they felt about the choice to specialize in palliative care at times like this. Smiling, Dr. Mohit said other kinds of specialists talk about life, but all palliative care specialists think about is death.

The conversation shifted back to Dr. Nigam, as it often did in the pain ward. Dr. Arjun marveled at how she survived death after death among her patients: "She's a very emotional person, and yet she has been doing this for twelve years now!" Often, they would describe her as a *bhavishyavan* (a divinator). Kamini (the patient who had just passed away) had come into the outpatient clinic a few days earlier. No other specialist at AIIMS had prognosticated how quickly her condition would decline; others had told her she still had time to live. At the outpatient clinic, I was told, Dr. Nigam had looked at Kamini and, after a brief examination, whispered to the residents that she had about three days to live and that they should immediately admit her to the inpatient ward to manage her pain. I had not been present when Dr. Nigam had prognosticated Kamini's death in the way that had struck the residents, but I had seen many times before how she and other more experienced palliative care residents quickly took in the condition of patients even in the most fleeting of outpatient clinic encounters.

These prognostic moments resisted formalization and verbalization in much the same way I described Dr. Arjun's tactile diagnosis of pain. Acutely ill palliative care patients presented with innumerable symptoms such as pain, anorexia, constipation, numbness, anxiety, difficulty swallowing, weakness, labored breathing, nausea, and insomnia. To complicate matters further, their etiologies and prognostic implications were as numerous as the symptoms themselves. The weakened bodies of cancer patients manifested pain and discomfort in unpredictable sites and ways, sometimes unrelated to the original tumors and malignancies and reflecting systemic bodily breakdowns. Dr. Nigam's ability to separate out the immediately life-threatening from the chronic was a skill she had developed through years of experience. In acute cases like Kamini's, she looked for subtle shifts in heart rate and pulse, the color and clamminess of the skin, shifts in the quality of breath, the manifestations of fatigue in the eyes and body language, the sites of pain and weakness, sensory amplification and numbness, and, always, the distribution of pain. She also would look for signs of delirium or visible distress. Because psychological distress is an inevitable consequence of a cancer diagnosis, she would have to distinguish the kinds of disturbance (dysphoria, hypomania, hallucinations, somnolence) and determine whether they were the side effects of drugs or instead indications of temporary bodily imbalance or significant organ failure. The expertise of prognostication rested on the reading of such subtle and constantly shifting signs, and a practiced ability to interpret them as a side effect of debilitating treatments or as a sign of permanent bodily breakdown.

On this last day of Kamini's life, the residents had tried to reach Dr. Nigam on the phone; she had been giving a lecture elsewhere in the city. Soon, Dr. Nigam arrived in visible distress at the residents' office. She was troubled not only because she had not been present at the time of death but also because the patient had not been sent home to be with her family. The residents apologetically explained that it had all happened quickly, and that the patient did not have an oxygen cylinder at home. Instead, they had brought the family to the ward to be with her in her last moments. I witnessed then how the inpatient ward had been turned into a space of grief, with curtains drawn, doors closed, and the family at the side of the patient. As silence fell upon this conversation, we could hear Kamini's husband weeping in the corridor between the office and the inpatient ward. Dr. Nigam tidied herself up and walked out to him. Through the doorway, I watched her standing with her arm on his shoulder, letting him cry. In a sight that was rare elsewhere in the hospital, I saw a doctor and patient grieving together in a space that for a moment felt less like a hospital and more like a place of mourning.

If relating to pain produced demands of empathy and recognition, witnessing death produced resonant claims. If pain attuned physicians to the limits of their interventions to ease suffering, witnessing death dramatized a similar helplessness in the face of human mortality. This reminder shook Dr. Arjun, even after his tumor turned out to be benign. The same reminder hung over Dr. Mohit, even as he struggled against all odds to save his father's life. The possibility of death was an ever-present haunting at the palliative care ward. In a hospital space designed to save or at least maintain life, the palliative care ward marked a zone where life could be allowed to ebb away. In 2013, Dr. Nigam wrote a powerful piece that captures this paradox. The piece began with her consoling a senior resident drained by her repetitive confrontation with death. This encounter pushed Dr. Nigam to ask: "All through as a medical student, we were preparing her to fight death, the enemy. We never prepared her to face the inevitable truth that death is a part of life. I pondered who really is afraid of death, the patient or us?" Growing out of this question, her hope for the medical profession was that it "accept death as an essential friend of all life forms, not a foe." If confronting pain demanded an acknowledgment of biomedicine's limits, confronting death demanded similar humility.

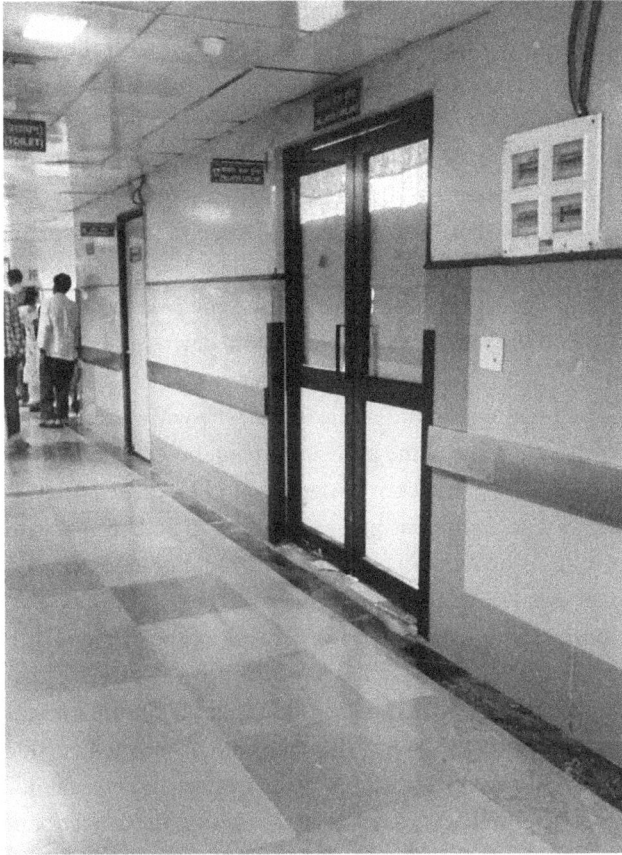

FIGURE 3.8
The palliative care
unit at AIIMS, with
its door closed.
Photo by author.

The Bounds of Empathy

The exceptionality of the space of the palliative care ward and the practices of empathy that were produced in its midst cannot be exaggerated. The perception in India that Dr. Arjun referred to—of doctors as uncaring and rude to patients from lower socioeconomic strata—is an enduring accusation, and not without some truth. Toward the end of my fieldwork, an investigative television show dramatically reenacted countless horrors perpetrated on patients by greedy doctors. At the same time, a study was being conducted at a nearby tertiary care hospital in Delhi. The study concluded that about 40 percent of doctors reported experiencing violence in the previous year, because of patients who were furious and frustrated by what they imagined to be medical negligence.[55] By the time of my last follow-up visits to AIIMS, I found that the institute had begun to offer self-defense martial arts lessons to its medical staff, to guard against patients who turned against them. The careful practices of empathy I have described here contrast with these accusations of malpractice and neglect and a perception of unfeeling doctors pushing patients to their death.

A few years after my fieldwork, I found such accusations recur in a different register in a piece written by Sumegha Gulati, a journalist for *The Caravan* magazine. This was her "last dispatch" written for the magazine as she struggled with cancer.[56] In these writings, Gulati described the suffocating crowds within the cancer hospital at AIIMS. She recalled how her father would have to join the registration queue before dawn for every chemotherapy session, since only patients who registered by eight o'clock in the morning would receive treatment. While inside, she witnessed several confrontations between guards and the patients' attendants seeking a word with their doctors. Each day, at least ten patients would be turned away at night, as time ran out for accommodating even those who had been able to register in the morning. When Gulati's cancer recurred, her experience at AIIMS motivated her to move to Bombay for treatment.

If Gulati—an upper-class journalist with a network of social support in the city—described her experience as "harrowing," it is no surprise that poorer patients who often travel long distances to reach the hospital might be at an even further end of their tether. Talking to patients queued outside the hospital, I heard endless angry accounts of prior neglect and present duress. One patient I spoke to stated that he was only visiting the cancer pain clinic because he was leaving for his home in Bihar the next day. The oncologist had told him his tumor needed to be surgically excised. He had heard too many stories of unnecessary surgeries in government hospitals, and he had no interest in being experimented on. He hoped that the clinic might give him enough morphine to afford him a couple of pain-free weeks back at his village. When I cautiously suggested this might be the wrong course of action, he shot back that people lost limbs and body parts at hospitals all the time against their will. Accusations of such medical malpractice are pervasive in India, and AIIMS has not been exempt. In 2007, a consumer court found AIIMS liable for the unnecessary mastectomy of a woman wrongly diagnosed with cancer. The next year the hospital was forced to set up an internal committee to review the death of a thirty-five-year-old man who had died when his oxygen mask was removed while he was being wheeled into the cancer institute. Rumors, investigations, and charges such as these have done little to bolster the credibility of public cancer care.

Palliative care unfolds in Delhi in the shadow of these widespread perceptions of medical neglect, corruption, and malpractice. If I found that on-cologists in the cancer hospital often withdrew from engaging with patients after terminal prognoses, I saw how it fell upon pain and palliative care specialists to deal with the last weeks of a patient's life. Thus, the pain clinic came to stand in as the space of hope for dying well, the provisional rubrics of a compassionate response to those who had been denied timely treatment. Yet, this is not to say that the care Kamini and Hardeep received was repre-sentative of treatment at the pain clinic. Dr. Arjun was not being overly self-critical when he said he could not help but shout at many patients under his care. Nor were all patients as demanding of their right to care as Hardeep. But while he would sometimes lose his temper, Dr. Arjun worked well over the institute's mandated forty-hour workweek, as did his colleagues. His eight-hour workday inevitably stretched to twelve, and sometimes longer if there was a patient in particular distress. It was within these conditions of infrastructural pressure that the palliative care team sought to treat and al-leviate cancer pain.

How might we best understand the contours and limits of empathy in these conditions of both care and disregard at the cancer hospital? Through-out this chapter, I have described the trajectories and orientations of empa-thy that came to be improvised in this space that demanded the recognition of pain and the inevitability of death. Palliative care research—in its quest for transcendence—sought to respond and ease the existential distress that was partly an outcome of a debilitating disease, and partly a consequence of these infrastructural pressures and lacks. In so doing, it looked to available vocabularies to formulate pathways through which pain could be dispersed and diffused. An appeal to transcendence offered one way out, a way to look past the dispiriting conditions of everyday failures and toward the resilient capacities of a mind strengthened by the development of its spiritual ca-pacities. In practice, however, palliative care physicians took another tack. The rubrics of empathy that were taught and transacted in the work of rec-ognizing pain emphasized an acknowledgment of limits. If pain remained intractable, empathy involved an attunement to intractability, while main-taining therapeutic relations as far into the illness as possible. Thus, on the one hand, the recognition of suffering entailed transcendence; on the other, it required a grappling with limits.

At the same time, while research and practice diverged on the forms of recognition and practices of empathy, the two forms of palliative care work shared an underlying limit. Both research and practice enlarged what cancer pain encapsulated, mobilizing the biomedical specialty's imaginations of the "psychosocial." Both research and practice produced responsive modes of feeling, empathy, and recognition that allowed for interventions into easing and ameliorating this pain. But in these same gestures, biomedical palliative care practitioners stopped short of an even more expansive vision, one that could include the structural preconditions of pain that were a result of long-standing public health failures. For all the provisional possibilities of empathy and recognition, palliative care remained trapped within the institutional failures that characterize public health care in India.

Even after decades of pioneering work, Dr. Nigam too expressed dissatisfaction with the pace at which her field was developing. In a reflective piece on the discipline published in 2015, she wrote that a "lack of acknowledgment of people's suffering, lack of acceptance of a separate medical specialty and apathy are largely responsible for the unheard agony and preventable suffering thriving even five decades after the big bang origin of the modern hospice and palliative care movement." She urged "sensitizing" the Indian medical and social worlds to the suffering of cancer patients. But, despite her frustrations, Dr. Nigam's mission to alleviate cancer pain continues unabated. Both before and after my fieldwork, in 2009 and then in 2018, newspapers covered her declaration that AIIMS would soon be transformed into a "pain-free" zone. In gestures such as these, Dr. Nigam displaced public health failures in treating cancer onto a more manageable project of at least relieving the institute's cancer patients from pain. The forms of recognition and empathy I have described throughout this chapter remain caught within this bind. The gestures that strive to recognize pain and suffering have little to say about the structural conditions that produce pain and suffering in the first place. Luc Boltanski describes the contemporary politics of empathy as that which "is not put into action in wholly general terms but is inscribed in particular relationships between particular individuals . . . an unfortunate whose suffering manifests itself locally."[57] The palliative care practice of seeing through the patients' eyes instantiated precisely such a model of empathy and recognition. In highlighting the immediacy and urgency of pain, practitioners were forced to push aside questions of health care justice and structural failures. These are, then, both the limits and the possibilities of the ethical commitment of palliative cancer care to "see through the patient's eyes," and the complexities of its mission to help the poor die free of pain.

4

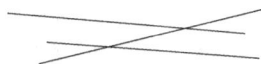

CANCER MEMOIRS

In the first two chapters of this book, cancer seemed to be a disease in search of a language, its everyday practices caught between speech and concealment. However, the aesthetic accounts I now turn to evidence no such reluctance to explicate the disease. In this and the next chapter, I examine memoirs and films about cancer produced in India. I do so because examining these accounts reveals a tension between the lived experience of cancer (that I have described so far) and its aesthetic representations. If in previous chapters I described a striving in everyday life to open spaces of indeterminacy, of inhabiting an irresolute "as-if," most aesthetic accounts of cancer resolve the ethical crises the disease produces in social life. In other words, many of the memoirs and films I describe offer a way out of cancer's impasse. Sometimes they magnify the concerns of the disease onto the concerns of the nation, circumventing the problem by changing its scale. At other times, they urge patients to transcend the disease by a sheer force of personal will. And in yet other instances, they encourage patients to aspire toward a joyous postcancer future by expiating past sins that might have contributed to their disease. In these and many other ways, these aesthetic accounts offer ethical restitutions to their protagonists, at the same time offering clear lessons that might be learned from an encounter with the disease. In juxtaposing my fieldwork in previous chapters with these aesthetic accounts, I set up a contrast between the essential irresolution of my ethnographic narratives and its imagined resolvability in the written and filmic imagination. This juxtaposition of resolution with irresolvability, of restitution with skepticism, serves to sharpen my ethnographic description. In this chapter specifically, I focus on cancer memoirs written by patients after the turn of the century; in the next chapter, I examine Hindi films in the Indian postcolonial period that have taken cancer as their theme.

The Joy of Cancer

As a popular and recognizable genre, cancer memoirs came into their own in Europe and the United States around the 1960s. The Indian cancer memoir has a shorter history, gaining prominence in the early 2000s. These works most often are authored by patients who survive the disease, and less frequently by their near kin and caregivers. Most appear in one of four major Indian languages—English, Hindi, Marathi, and Kannada. Along with a corpus of other popular fiction, cancer memoirs, which usually are modestly priced, costing from about 30 to 200 rupees, are part of a vast production of popular literature intended primarily for a literate, indigenous audience. In this, they are far removed from the transnational literary worlds of globally recognized authors such as Salman Rushdie, Amitav Ghosh, Jhumpa Lahiri, and Arundhati Roy. While those more highbrow books are published by a few elite international and national presses, the cancer memoirs I discuss here are often self-published or produced in small runs by small local presses.

Most of these memoirs have the following formulaic structure. If the memoir is authored by a patient, that person is among the first to have received the diagnosis. As it is communicated, the diagnosis carries recrimination and blame. For example, the disclosure of the diagnosis to women in these memoirs is almost always accompanied by an accusation of self-neglect. In one account, the first question that a male doctor asks while revealing the diagnosis is, "How long have you known about the lump?," followed by an accusation: "Did you not check yourself regularly?" Such accusations are described by memoirists without criticizing or commenting on the doctor's approach. For example, the writer who received these accusations dedicated the book to the doctor who made them, describing him without irony as a paragon of sensitivity. In another account, a young memoirist in her thirties strikes up a conversation with a female doctor while receiving her mammogram. She tells her doctor she was surprised to discover her lump because she was told that the diagnosis was unlikely before the age of forty. In response, the doctor accuses her of lying to evade blame for her own failure in detecting the lump earlier.[1] When the mammogram confirms a cancer diagnosis, the doctor refuses to talk to the patient, since she has already demonstrated herself as incapable of personal responsibility, and asks that her husband be brought in. In another account, a writer recalls that while communicating her diagnosis, her doctors told her that her cancer was a manifestation of her unresolved grief for her husband's recent death.[2] In yet another, the memoirist—a botany professor—is similarly assailed for ignoring her symptoms; her doctor tells her that cancer in India was a recent problem brought on by "modernity" and "urban multitasking women" who ignored their own symptoms were partially responsible for its epidemic outbreak. This linked accusation recurs in many such memoirs: that cancer was a new disease brought on by contemporary unhealthy lifestyles, and that women who had entered the workforce were not entirely undeserving victims. For much of the book, the professor-memoirist grapples with this accusation. Toward the end, she breaks down and admits that she had been "foolish, illiterate and ignorant" in trying to pursue her career and care for her family at the same time.[3] Like many others, she expresses gratitude for her physician's acute insight. However, this internalization of blame is not without cognitive dissonance. The patient oscillates between feeling guilty about her "selfishness" and taking pride in her work as a professional.

While women face the brunt of moral recriminations, men too sometimes look to their past to find clues of moral failings. Men diagnosed with lung cancer were particularly prone to such reevaluations of their pasts. For example, the disease pushes one author to reexamine his karmic credit and debts.[4] Anup Kumar seeks a guru who urges him to think about how he might prevent its transmission to his children. Understanding karma as a matter of self-responsibility for the past, he feels an urgent need to remove any hatred for his own cancer, since hatred leads to the accumulation of "evil karma." He takes for granted a cultural truism—"some say" cancer is self-imposed—assuming one incurs cancer by gathering resentments. The solution to this lies in self-acceptance, without which any kind of treatment is bound to fail. Men's self-reevaluations differ slightly from women's in that they are rarely forced by accusations and blame. Their past misdeed is not that they neglected familial care—a domain reserved for women to worry about. Rather, their self-reflections show they retain their penchant for intellectualism, despite the disease.

A period of shock follows this revelation, when the memoir's main protagonist—either kin or patient—is thrown into despair, disbelief, anger, or delirium and withdraws from social life. But this withdrawal can only be temporary; the demands of treatment and kinship responsibilities require a reentry into interpersonal relations. This raises other questions: Whom should they tell, and from whom should they hide the diagnosis? In memoirs authored by patients, they are often the first to know: doctors tell some, while others find out from kin. But if the memoir is authored by a family member, disclosure is trickier. Even when the patient or kin are doctors, the first impulse is always to keep the diagnosis secret and prevent the psychic harm brought on by its communication.[5] This is not the only argument offered in favor of secrecy. Often, neighbors appear not as helpful allies but as vindictive aggravators of a patient's distress. One memoirist recounts how a neighbor asked her to make charitable contributions to wash away sins from previous lifetimes, leading her to feel like the "biggest sinner on the planet."[6] Two other memoirists remember neighbors arriving at their homes to tell them harrowing stories of the painful deaths of other cancer patients. To make a diagnosis public invites such possibilities of accusation, convincing most to keep their cancer secret.

While adjusting to life after diagnosis, patients and kin are faced with the difficult choice between public and private treatment. If the protagonists are not wealthy, they worry about the decrepit state of public hospitals, where, for the first time, they will rub shoulders with the country's poorest. For some, these visits lead to reflections about socioeconomic inequality. One account describes the shock thus: "A sudden sense of depression set in me as we saw patients there: many looked emaciated; those who had enlarged lymph glands were seen with their glands projecting downwards . . . some had fixed blank stares." For most memoirists, these sights are enough to drive them away from public hospitals and toward expensive private facilities, even at potentially catastrophic financial cost. For others, this encounter with poverty provides an opportunity for a new empathetic orientation toward the poor. One memoirist writes: "Never had I seen so many maimed and bruised specimens of humanity. . . . There were people who had been cut open, stitched, and were waiting. . . . Surprisingly, not once did I hear anybody cursing life or fate. . . . All I saw was the incongruity of dignified acceptance."[7] She is then amazed to find love among these scenes of suffering: "Did I actually see more rural, down-to-earth people, as opposed to the busy professionals of the metros, living out true love?" After much rumination about the nature of love, she recommends: "Whoever you are, whatever age you are, you do deserve to make a trip to this hospital at once. You need to feel first-hand, the heartbreak of patients being abandoned by their own or the sheer joy of a son looking after his widowed mother. . . . You *must* experience raw human drama present itself in the corridors here."[8] She returns home not disillusioned or terrified but delighted by such instructive scenes of resilience and love.

For those not inspired by such scenes of suffering, privatized care shows the failure of public care. For example, Kamlesh Tripathi—a self-described "corporate citizen"—tells the story of his son Shravan, who died after fourteen years of living with brain cancer. In the memoir, Shravan asks his father about where the money for his expensive medicine comes from. Tripathi replies that the corporation he works for pays for it. Shravan then asks whether Tripathi has thanked them for their help. The memoir fulfills Shravan's request and is as much a panegyric to the corporation that employed Tripathi as it is a story of Shravan's cancer. Always grateful for privatized care, only once does Tripathi wonder about those who do not enjoy corporate philanthropy, asking, what is the "medical business model for the poor?"[9]

Some memoirs detail the debilitating effects of their author's cancer treatments, but usually descriptions of such vulnerability are quickly transcended. In a telling phrase, one writer describes her pain as "only the pain of rebirth."[10] Treatment offers an opportunity to find joy, love, and victory. This is the most important lesson of the Indian cancer memoir: that pain is the precondition for transcendence. The centrality of this theme in the memoirs is evidenced by their titles: *The Joy of Cancer, Not Out: Winning the Game of Cancer, Cancer Made Me, To Cancer, with Love, My Date with Cancer*, and so on. Mimicking the structure of revelation common in self-help books, these memoirs arrive at a climactic conclusion that one might not only survive cancer but also find a more authentic self in recovery. This victory offers a further insight: that good health is a matter of belief and will. For example, in one memoir an author seeks to dispel common myths about cancer in India; the myth that "being positive will cure cancer" occupies a prominent place in the list. However, instead of counteracting this myth, she confirms it. She writes that a positive outlook not only makes the disease more bearable but also "determines the efficacy of medicine," since "ultimately, it is all in your mind."[11] Thus, the centrality of the theme of positivity is most apparent when even an effort to dispel it compels a contrary admission: "So, in the larger sense of the term, one may say that being positive will help cure your cancer." Empowered by their new sense of mental fortitude at having faced and escaped death, most writers look forward to a life filled with optimism and positivity.

The same gesture that promises a joyful future also refigures the past.

FIGURE 4.1
Cover image from
The Joy of Cancer,
a memoir by Anup
Kumar.

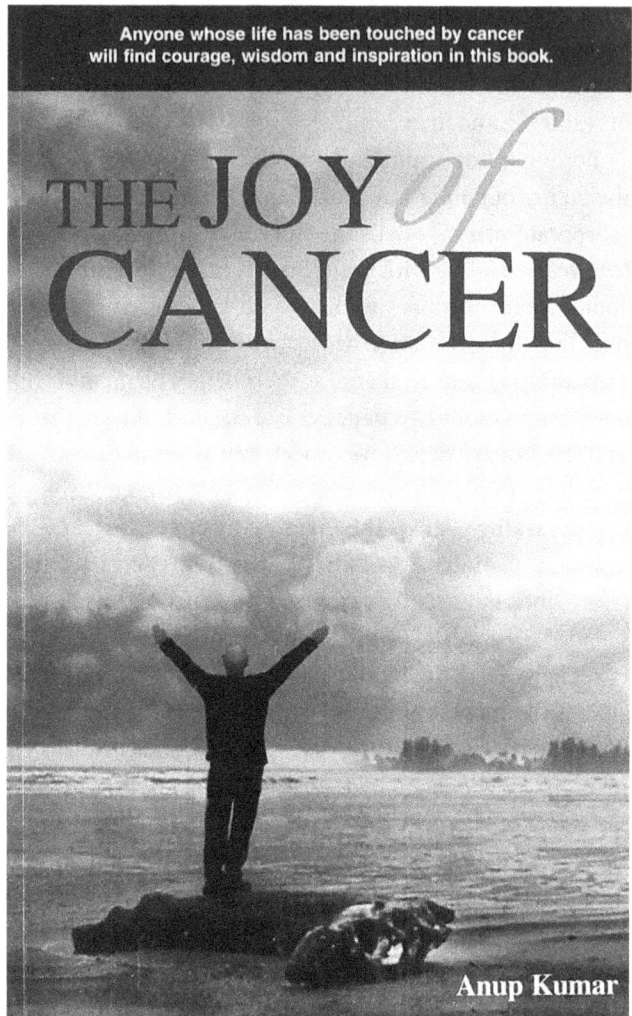

Anyone whose life has been touched by cancer will find courage, wisdom and inspiration in this book.

THE JOY *of* CANCER

Anup Kumar

The patient's depressive personality at an earlier time in life is understood as having contributed to the disease. While not a memoir, one of the most successful self-help books on cancer focuses on the harmful effects of a patient's inclination toward depression.[12] It is one of the few popular books on cancer that has consistently remained in print in India and found a global audience. Its author, Dr. Nitin Unkule, has spoken to audiences at the World Health Organization and cancer hospitals all over the world. In his book, Unkule takes credit for the discovery of a "cancer personality" as the disease's etiology. Never mind that the idea of a cancer personality has been a cultural trope in the United States at least since the 1960s, when the first medical

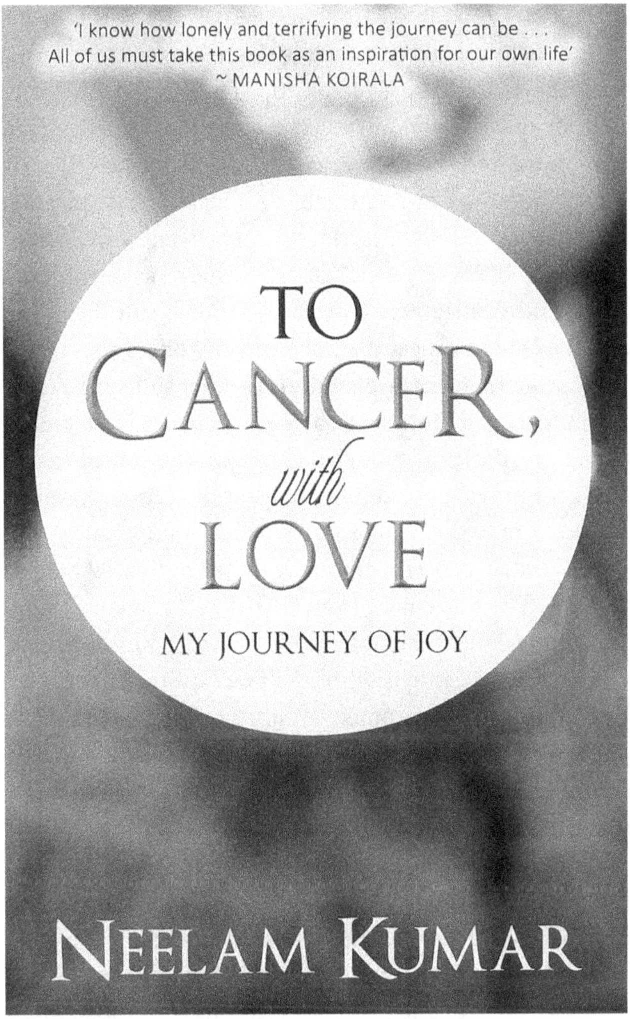

FIGURE 4.2
Cover image from
To Cancer, with Love,
a memoir by Neelam
Kumar.

'I know how lonely and terrifying the journey can be . . .
All of us must take this book as an inspiration for our own life'
~ MANISHA KOIRALA

TO
CANCER,
with
LOVE

MY JOURNEY OF JOY

NEELAM KUMAR

studies sought to test the hypothesis that maladaptive personalities contributed to cancer.[13] But this does not stop Unkule. He divides cancer patients
into two groups—survivors, who have peace of mind, and "diers," who are
full of denial and depression. There is no such thing as incurable cancer,
Unkule suggests, only incurable patients. To lend his ideas a veneer of scientific credibility, he describes "cancer phantom" cells that he knows about,
but that "the West" has yet to discover. Predictably, if patients are to blame
for their cancer, Unkule suggests, they must take responsibility for their own
cure. Such a cure is only possible if patients acknowledge their own blame
and set out to live a new life full of optimism and cheer. Although not a

memoir, Unkule's book makes clear the troubling telos of the cancer memoir, if its mantras of self-help are taken to their logical end.

What might we make of the generic conventions of the Indian cancer memoir? What kinds of affective identifications are promised to readers in these journeys from blame and shock to recovery and recuperation? Certainly, these memoirs summon an intimate public—a space of identification between strangers that Lauren Berlant describes as coemergent with popular print culture.[14] Her phrase "intimate public" describes many mass-produced cultural forms that promise consumers they are not alone, that their pain is shared by others. The Indian cancer memoir similarly offers a seductive possibility of identification. In its mode of address to other suffering cancer patients, the form presupposes an intimacy based on the fact of a shared illness. But at the same time, these memoirs bear the paradox at the heart of all intimate publics. They provide possibilities of emotional contact even as such contact presupposes only the thinnest grounds of commonality. Authors and readers of the Indian cancer memoir are united by the fact of their diagnosis, and little else. The movement from "I" to "we," fundamental to the form of address of the cancer memoir, articulates a common vulnerability to illness, but it rests on an elision of the practical nature of these vulnerabilities. In other words, the promise of intimacy in these memoirs is predicated on obscuring how social differences such as class and gender structure differential access to survival and recovery. There is little proximal support in such promises of cancer publics.

At the same time, such a transcendence of social complexity is more than a precondition for fictive intimacies around cancer; it is also its reward. Join us, the memoirist promises, and learn the truth that cancer is not the curse it appears to be, but a path to a better, optimistic future. Such a promise is suffused with an unmistakable cruelty.[15] To arrive at this revelation and its promise of a "good life," protagonists must look away from the obstacles that hinder their flourishing. Patriarchal accusations of self-neglect must be accepted and internalized, class hierarchies are pushed to the narrative margin, and the fantasy of recovery hides the danger that cancer might recur. Dangerously, then, this unfettered optimism not only promises a disease-free future but also does little to prepare for the possibility that such a future might be interrupted. Accusations of neglect might return, financial distress might again force the difficult choice between public and private care, decisions about disclosure might again have to be made. But for the promise of transcendence to be plausible, cancer—the very object that throws life into jeopardy—becomes a peculiar object of desire and attachment. Again, memoir titles most transparently reveal this paradox: cancer is a "lover," a "date," the protagonist's "maker," and the source of future "joy." Thus, the conventional premise of the Indian cancer memoir is that cancer not only allows the opportunity to recover life but also serves as a precondition for *having* a life. There is no space here for grief, for the paradox that endurance and survival come at difficult social costs, or for the possibility that life might be lived in the irresolute space of its debris.

Against Restitution

So far, I have described the Indian cancer memoir in its most conventional form. As such, the genre offers little reflection on the darker corners of the disease. There is no space here for a statement such as literary theorist Kathlyn Conway's that, after two decades with the illness, "the experience of cancer is without redeeming value; that I have not been transformed by the experience; that it is, beyond all else, a misery to be endured."[16] Conway is allied with a select group of memoirists—including Arthur Frank and Reynolds Price—who reflect on the limits of the genre and critique its "restitution narrative" from health, to sickness, and back to health.[17] The expression "restitution narratives" aptly describes the Indian cancer memoirs I have discussed, and my analysis of them has been informed by Conway and others who express discomfort with how Euro-American cancer memoirs often ally disease with redemption. At the same time, Conway holds on to the hope that the cancer memoir might be rescued from itself. For writers and critics in Conway's mold, the way out of this generic impasse is to confront the messy fact of death and grapple with what Price calls in his own memoir the "far side of catastrophe."[18] Through writing, Conway hopes to recover the ability to give illness meaning as that most "utterly human process" and death as that most "basic human condition."[19] Through this direct confrontation with the possibility of death and life's unraveling, the genre's most reflexive writers hope to rescue it from disrepute.

In what follows I describe similar efforts in India that seek to escape the limitations of this genre. In this, I join critics like Conway who hope to recover cancer narratives from their seemingly self-evident association with the tropes of self-help. Reflecting on her critical literary practice while grappling with her husband's cancer, Ann Jurecic argues that a suspicion toward such narratives risks a disengagement with what aesthetic genres might offer to those who live with critical illness.[20] My way of remaining open to the promise of aesthetic accounts of the disease is to foreground those that hesitate in their search for narrative resolution and restitution. Certainly, some of the cancer memoirs I have described so far reproduce the same unsatisfying narratives of personal growth and willed transcendence that have drawn justifiable scholarly ire elsewhere in the world. At the same time, the ones I will now go on to describe depart from this trope, portraying practices of endurance that rarely resolve in easy recovery and restitution. These accounts offer multiple, fragmented, and even contradictory accounts of everyday life with the disease. In remaining partial and incomplete, they offer a more faithful picture of the irresolvable contradictions that living and dying with the illness produces.

Even though my impulse here might resemble that of scholars like Conway who encourage attentiveness to the "universal" and "basic" fact of life's unraveling, I depart from their method in one important regard. Conway's aim, reflected in many excellent accounts of cancer in recent years, is to get past the injunction to hope against all odds and instead to confront the messy, human, and universal fact of death that haunts all human experience.[21] Such efforts hope to remind biomedical patients and practitioners increasingly obsessed with extending life that "death, of course, is not a failure. Death is normal . . . the natural order of things."[22] On the other hand, my effort here is to understand how certain memoirs explore the contingency of death not as a "human" or "universal" question but as an entryway into asking what it means to live and die rooted in a *particular* time and place. In other words, in confronting the solitude that might accompany a cancer diagnosis, these works articulate an estrangement from living within *a* world, rather than *the* world in some universal, abstract sense. Here, the lines between this and the far side of catastrophe are not defined by whether or not the memoirist can confront the fact of human mortality. Rather, the lines dividing the ordinary from the catastrophic can loosen and tighten in relation to specific arrangements of everyday life. The three memoirs I now turn to do not take a sense of the catastrophic as a universal human lesson. Rather, their sense of the catastrophic grows out of experiences of everyday lives rooted in the vicissitudes of specific histories.

Nazeem Beegum's memoir, *My Mother Did Not Go Bald*, includes an introduction by the Malayalam writer Maythil Radhakrishnan.[23] What commends the book to Radhakrishnan is Beegum's rejection of a restitutive authorial voice. The book's chapters are titled "Bystanders 1" through "Bystanders 22," with each bystander representing a different aspect of Beegum's self, fragmented into these different pieces after her mother's cancer diagnosis. In that single stylistic gesture, Beegum allows the sediments of social de-

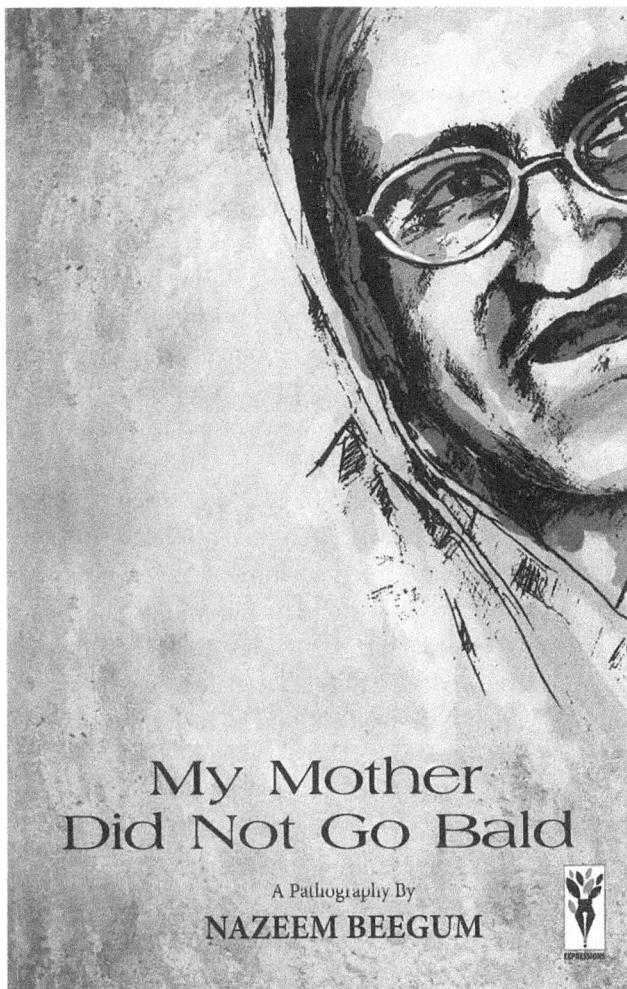

FIGURE 4.3 Cover image from *My Mother Did Not Go Bald*, a memoir by Nazeem Beegum.

bris in the wake of a cancer diagnosis to lodge into the book's form. As a "bystander," she struggles with a sense of powerlessness as her mother's cancer grows and metastasizes. She does not learn to "love" her mother's cancer, nor does she emerge as a victorious survivor after a battle with the disease. Instead, she is a witness, often silent, and almost always helpless. Each bystander—aspects of Beegum's fragmented self—bears witness, then, to how the disease puts pressure on already tense social ties.

The first relation that is tested is that between Beegum's mother—Ithata—and her brother. The book begins with Ithata asking to be sent home for a week from a palliative care ward. Her doctors understand this request as indicative of her desire to spend her last days at home, but Beegum senses a different motive: Ithata wants to go home to prepare her will and, through it, tempt her estranged son to return and see her. Even though Ithata's affection for her disloyal son upsets Beegum, she swallows her disappointment, acknowledging her mother's desire to repair her familial ties before her death. Ithata, too, recognizes how her continued loyalty to her son might make Beegum—an unselfish caregiver—feel devalued. To spare Beegum's feelings, she never explicitly expresses affection toward her son, instead offering practical pretexts for his return. But Ithata's plan to tempt her son back to her faces an obstacle. Various religious communities in India may legislate matters of marriage, divorce, and inheritance; Beegum and Ithata are Muslim, and their property transactions thus follow the guidelines of Muslim personal law. While Muslim personal laws in India are not strictly codified, they are usually interpreted in favor of male heirs, who get the larger shares of inheritances. Consequently, Ithata's son is not lured by her promise of an even larger share; he is satisfied with the property that will accrue to him with no performance of filial regard. Hurt by her son's disregard, Ithata returns to the palliative care ward, which happens to be run by Dr. Rajagopal, the preeminent name in palliative care in South India. In keeping with the palliative care injunction to bring quiescence to the dying patient, Dr. Rajagopal intervenes to resolve the family dispute. But Ithata's son refuses to come, even at Dr. Rajagopal's request.

While the familial bond that is most strained in Ithata's world is with her son, Beegum also describes how the diagnosis seeps into relations with other kin. Before Ithata's diagnosis, her sister had eloped with a man from another religion; now, she returns to ask for Ithata's forgiveness. Ithata forgives her, much to Beegum's dismay. Beegum blames her aunt for having put their family in jeopardy and wants her to continue to suffer the consequences of her actions. Again, Beegum is hurt by Ithata's gestures toward restituting her social ties. In describing this damage, Beegum allows us to glimpse unintended acts of violence that restitution can bring upon others in the same relational world. At the same time, Ithata's efforts at reconciliation come up against their own limits. In the last days of her life, Ithata prays in a room where another sister took her own life. She breaks down in this space, unable to understand how her sister could have ended her life, leaving broken social relations in her wake.

In another departure from the cheery optimism of restitution narratives, Beegum details Ithata's insistence on confronting her own mortality despite the best efforts of her kin to shield her from it. Beegum's sister is particularly adamant about not revealing Ithata's diagnosis to her. To this end, the family takes Ithata for treatment at a private hospital, even though this is beyond their financial means. Private hospitals are often enclosed in a single building, without clear signage dividing specialties from each other. The family hopes that this absence of explicit signposting in private hospitals—inescapable in public hospitals—would prevent Ithata from finding out she has cancer. However, their visit to the hospital coincides with World Cancer Day, and the hospital is dotted with banners picturing bald cancer patients. Beegum's sister is doubly upset when the oncologist at the hospital lets slip the word "biopsy" in Ithata's presence. They realize afterward that Ithata knew more than she let on; while leaving the hospital, she asks them if they noticed the banners and signs. Still, they keep up the pretense of secrecy and never talk about the diagnosis, even as it haunts many of their conversations. But closer to her death, Ithata again forces an acknowledgment of her cancer and its terminal prognosis. She asks to see her *kafan*—the ritual cloth and perfumes in which she will be buried. This request troubles Beegum, and she puts it off. Ithata dies the next day, leaving Beegum with the guilt of having denied her mother her last wish.

In its acknowledgment of fragmentation, grief, and mortality, *My Mother Did Not Go Bald* fulfills the ambitions of many scholarly and literary critics for cancer memoirs. It does so not only by confronting death but also by grappling with what dying means in a particular time and place. That is, the book reverberates with the specific arrangements of kinship, gender, and voice that are not "universal" or "basic," as Conway would have it, but deeply rooted in social worlds. These twin felicities of the book—its acknowledgment of mortality and the descriptions of its contextual specificity—come together in the final metaphor of the kafan. Anthropologists have long argued that funeral arrangements, both pre- and postmortem, are a way for social actors to resolve the personal and social ruptures resulting from death and grief.[24] While gesturing to its possibility, Beegum rejects this resolution. The funeral itself becomes another symbol for unresolved grief, and a site of frustration and helplessness for Beegum.

Mayan, a Hindi memoir, echoes the entanglement of kinship and illness in *My Mother Did Not Go Bald*, but it reaches a remarkably different conclusion.[25] Written by novelist Anand Prakash Maheshwari, it tells the story of his mother's cancer. Maheshwari seeks to put some distance between his life and writing and takes on the pseudonym Vineet through the course of the memoir. The book is named for the honorific—Mayan—by which Vineet addresses his mother. Mayan is diagnosed with cancer and is treated at the All India Center of Medical Sciences (AIIMS). In Vineet's account, she is the paragon of a selfless mother, who in times of familial poverty gave up her own food so that her children might eat; when food was especially scarce, she would eat it stale. Vineet traces the etiology of Mayan's cancer to this eating of stale food and to the overabundance of her piety and filial love. Humbled by her sacrifice, he sets about sacrificing himself to care for her. He regrets his careless life before Mayan's disease and is now resolved to become the dutiful son she deserves. His first sacrifice is to hide the diagnosis from her. This involves careful subterfuges that unravel as she enters AIIMS for treatment and reads the hospital signs. Through the course of his mother's illness, Vineet's desire to sacrifice himself grows, as does his impatience with others who disrupt his duty. He reserves his strongest condemnation for neighbors who, he reports, only exacerbate Mayan's distress by recounting the painful deaths of other cancer patients. As her disease progresses toward her death, he isolates her from all social contact other than his own.

Mayan is conflicted about Vineet's relentless need to sacrifice. It appears that a real source of concern for her is Vineet's growing anger against his father and his need to atone for his father's sins. Mayan and her husband are estranged, and the novel hints at the possibility of past domestic violence as the cause of this estrangement. To mitigate Vineet's anger against his father, Mayan reminds him of a story of her early marital life. When Mayan and her husband first lived together after marriage, social codes dictated that they would never directly address each other. Instead, they would always address each other via a third person, even while in each other's presence: "Please tell him that . . ." But once, when both were alone in their house for a few days, Mayan fell sick. This raised the problem of how Mayan could communicate with her husband and not break social taboos. To circumvent this problem, her husband would sleep just outside her door with a rope tied to his toe. The other end of the rope was near Mayan, who could tug it without calling his name. This entanglement of care with the violence that would soon overwhelm the marriage gives Vineet some respite from his resentment. It also gives pause to the narrative Vineet constructs about his mother's lifelong victimhood, which drives his desire to sacrifice himself at the altar of her deification.

But the pause is brief. The second half of the book takes place in a claustrophobic arrangement of Mayan and Vineet sequestered in the room where she will die. In the long hours he spends with her every day, he turns to the world of myth to bring Mayan solace. The book becomes an explicit mirror of an episode and its aftermath in the Mahabharata, specifically the passages now referred to as the Bhagavad Gita. In the myth, these passages appear in a battle between two groups of warring brothers. The Gita comprises a dialogue between the prince, Arjuna, and his divine charioteer, Krishna, during the battle. Seeing the devastation on the battlefield, Arjuna despairs at the consequences of war. In response, Krishna comes to his aid, convincing him to fulfill his duty as a warrior.[26] The memoir then takes the form of an ethical dialogue between Vineet and his mother, who talk for hours about theological doctrine and grapple with the ethics of suffering and death. As the book progresses, it shifts its reference point to a later episode in the Mahabharata that is the Gita's aftermath. The myth is of Bhishma, a warrior so powerful that Arjuna and Krishna can only stop him in battle with deception. After he is brought down, Bhishma lies between life and death on a bed of arrows that Arjuna lays down as a show of respect. Early in his life, Bhishma had been granted a boon that allowed him to determine the precise moment of his death. Invoking his boon, Bhishma lives in pain in the verge between life and death, steadfast in his desire to witness the conclusion of the war. For Vineet, Bhishma is the perfect analogue for Mayan's suffering. While Bhishma can choose the moment of his death, he cannot choose its cause or trajectory; those are determined by forces outside his control. As for Arjuna, all he can do is witness in despair the consequences of his ethical fulfillment. This episode in the Mahabharata is a fundamental moment of insight for Vineet. Inspired by it, he understands his own book as a minor meditation on the "art of dying." For weeks, Vineet and Mayan talk day and night about theology, myths, and what it might mean for her to die well. Near the end of her life, they decide to withdraw her morphine so that she may live out her karmic burden. This is Vineet's practical application of Bhishma's instructive ethical act to witness his own death despite the intense suffering of his body.

Mayan is a book that resists a straightforward gloss. Its many twists and turns allow for a plurality of insights that are rare in other accounts. In the time of self-help books on the art of living with and surviving cancer with cheery optimism, it is one of the few accounts of cancer that explores the "art of dying." It takes recourse simultaneously to myth, biomedicine, and the biographical pasts of its protagonists. Bhishma was given the boon of choosing the moment of his death so that he might die well: a self-willed death is fundamental to many theological conceptualizations in Hindu thought. However, this boon turns out to be inadequate to the task within the contexts of a war and the ethical demands of living in times of moral confusion.

The invocation of the Bhishma myth in *Mayan* is thus particularly apt. It reveals the narrative's acknowledgment of the limitations of arriving at a good death through a preordained set of prescriptions; there is no simple set of rituals, practices, and incantations that can conjure this into being for Mayan. Rather, the weight of the present and past—something Vineet glosses as a "karmic burden"—weighs on his account, blocking the possibility of resolution. The "art of dying" in the book, then, appears in the form of a dialogue that is conducted over days and nights, coaxing together various registers of the biomedical, mythic, and personal.

At the same time, the dialogue between Vineet and Mayan is really his monologue. The book's turn to the mythic eclipses the voice of the patient in pain. This elision of Mayan's voice is especially acute toward the end. As the disease's effects multiply, so does Vineet's desire to speak for her. We must strain to hear Mayan's presence in the book as it is increasingly overlaid by Vineet's ethical musings about her illness. Vineet's desire to reciprocate his mother's sacrifices with his own is overwhelming, enveloping both the narrative and the trajectory of Mayan's death. I find, then, that almost contrary to its author's intent, the book reveals the deep violence that the ethical single-mindedness of sacrifice metes out to vulnerable recipients, unable or unwilling to withstand its force. As much as Vineet might believe that his own sacrifice helps produce his mother's "good death," I read his actions as further silencing his already vulnerable mother, who is disallowed any agency in determining the trajectory of her dying. Nowhere is this more striking than in Vineet's insistence on taking away her analgesia so she may live out her "karmic burden." This ethical complexity of the relation between sacrifice, critical illness, and the violence of witnessing is one of the book's unintended but powerful insights.

So far in my readings of Indian cancer memoirs, I have been arguing that a precondition for a book exceeding generic conventions is its openness to narrative irresolution. While most accounts seek a transcendence of illness through the sheer force of optimism, some—*My Mother Did Not Go Bald* and *Mayan* among them—make more space for the possibility of death and the presence of grief. In such memoirs, cancer does not lead to an enumeration of new prescriptions for better living. Rather, they seek a structure of representation proper to the fragmentation of their world. At the same time, they do so in different ways and to different ends. If *My Mother Did Not Go Bald* leaves the fragmentation of grief unresolved, allowing it to become part of the book's structure, in *Mayan* the "art of dying" resolves such fragmentation through new injunctions to self-sacrifice and a mythos of ethical and redemptive suffering. I now turn to a third memoir—*Silent Echoes*—that opens another possibility of narrativizing the relation between fragmentation, redemption, and recovery. It describes how the experience of cancer reveals the contextually rooted fragilities of life that precede and follow a cancer diagnosis. When the disease enters its narrative, it marks not the beginning or end of a person's vulnerability but a new point of relational stress in a long biography of suffering.

Like *Mayan*, *Silent Echoes* blurs the lines between fiction and biography. Although it is presented as a memoir, the preface reveals that it was ghostwritten and that the subject of the memoir remains anonymous. The reason for this masking is that *Silent Echoes* tells a story of domestic violence that is still hidden from many of the author's acquaintances and kin. Its main protagonist, Prerna, grows up in India but is sent to England to be married. She does not know this when she arrives in the country, only finding out when her parents leave her there with her brother and return home. Despite this abandonment, she writes approvingly of "Indian society" and its adherence to the moral institution of the family. Within weeks, her marriage is arranged with a groom in a city close to where her brother lives in England. Prerna's marital abuse begins immediately after her marriage, motivated by her in-laws' dissatisfaction with the dowry they received from her family. She is sexually assaulted by her father-in-law, but she does not speak out so that she can live out her childhood dream of being married. She is constantly beaten by each of her in-laws—her husband, as well as his parents and his brother. She is disallowed personal possessions and forbidden from having contact with her natal kin. Even when she talks to her natal kin, she hides her abuse from them, hoping to spare them her suffering and the self-blame it might induce in them. Even after all this abuse, the cruelty of her optimism continues unabated. She becomes pregnant and gives birth, expecting the entry of a child into the family to quell the violence. In this, too, she is disappointed, and the violence continues after her son's birth. At this difficult biographical moment, Prerna is diagnosed with cancer.

Instead of drawing sympathy from those around her, Prerna's disease only exacerbates her vulnerability. Her in-laws want her out of their house, hoping she will die quietly with her natal kin. This hope is motivated by their desire for her husband's remarriage, which would be tainted if prospective families found out about her stigmatized disease. She lives with her brother but never gives up hope that her affinal family will take her back after she recovers. She tells her brother of her abuse, but they decide that divorce would bring shame on their family and that she should seek reconciliation. Prerna continues to blame herself and even considers suicide. She talks about pain as if it lives only in others and not in herself: for example, she worries endlessly about how it would anguish her kin if they found out about her suffering. And to communicate her pain to her husband, she slaps their son, to which her husband responds by beating her. She asks then that if he feels the pain in a baby so acutely, why can he not imagine the pain of her parents? Through the course of her treatments, Prerna's natal kin offer the support her affinal kin refuse. She is struck by the irony that they will protect her from the violence of cancer, but not of kinship. Slowly, her every certainty about her place in this world comes undone: "I knew that I was homeless. No one's home or rented place would ever become my home."[27] She realizes not only that her affinal kin will never take her back but also that her natal kin see her as a burden.

Yet, these realizations do not eclipse Prerna's hopes for marital reconciliation. She wishes, despite herself, that her husband will take her back once her hair grows back. The last fragments of her hope collapse only when she receives divorce papers from him. She writes then of the "fragmentation, isolation and meaningless" of suffering, realizing that her cancer offered her no pathway to a good life.[28] Finally, she is able to acknowledge her abandonment: "Even the killer disease did not free me from the shackles of culture. If it had been Sajan [her husband] having cancer, everyone would openly have asked me to look after him and do things in the best possible way to help him through the disease. However, no one really cared, no one looked at it that way for me."[29]

About this time, her sister is murdered by her own in-laws following a dowry dispute. Prerna knew her sister had an unhappy marriage. She had been born with a mole that had been surgically removed, but the scar hurt her marriage prospects, and she had been married to the first family that agreed to take her in. The murder of Prerna's sister proves to be the proverbial last straw. She absolves herself and her sister from blame for their own suffering and isolation. She writes that the history of women has been a history of silence, and that she would now revolt against this silence. But such a revolt turns out to involve something different from public testimony or an excision of her past. Her natal family helps her begin a career as a counselor, and she remains grateful to them. She remains close to her brother and sister, who are troubled that she chooses not to remarry. They see her unmarried state as a stigma that hurts their children's marriage prospects. Prerna does not bend under their pressure, but at the same time, she remains tied to them in bonds of both debt and affection.

Silent Echoes represents a remarkable exception to the Indian cancer memoir. Most tellingly, as with Ithata and Mayan, cancer enters Prerna's life through the troubled pathways of the violence in her past. As such, it offers no easy path to a new future freed from the shackles of past limits. The book refuses such an escape or transcendence. Even as she remakes herself during her recovery, Prerna remains entangled within her kinship obligations to her natal family. Instead of casting them off for not coming to her aid when she needed them, she continues to tend to these past ties. Her strategy, then, for living well in relation to destructive kinship norms is not to transcend them but to inhabit them differently. She leaves her violent affinal family but continues to respect their wish that she conceal her abuse. She chooses not to remarry but also lives with the accusation that this choice harms her family. In *Silent Echoes*, then, the past lives on in the present. Cancer bends but does not break kinship norms. The question of what it might mean to live well in the shadow of cancer thus appears only through an acknowledgment of the limits of recovery. Restitution cannot be understood here as a transcendence of past suffering through the new insights brought on by disease. Rather, understanding the force of cancer's violence requires Prerna to grapple with her marital past. The diagnosis does not catalyze new insight, marking a clean boundary between the past and present. Rather, it inflects certainties already under duress. And in this complex articulation of the past, present, and future, *Silent Echoes* allows a glimpse into a circumspect and plausible answer to the question of what it means to "survive" the violence of both gender and cancer, where the duress of one cannot be understood without reference to the other.

Against Optimism

On the surface, the cancer memoirs described in this chapter share the concerns of my face-to-face ethnographic work in prior chapters—how cancer enters and mutates social worlds. However, their explanations of this concern diverge from mine. During my fieldwork, I often found that for my ethnographic interlocutors, clear moral resolutions were never easily at hand. Nor was it possible to simply transcend the pain and duress of the disease by a sheer force of individual will. My ethnographic narratives reflect that indeterminacy, as well as the unfinished quality of my interlocutors' efforts to endure a cancer diagnosis. In most cancer memoirs, I found an opposite narrative orientation. Most looked past the fragility of social worlds within which the disease often appeared. They fled from the durable difficulties of everyday experience, instead offering stories of the joys of recovery and redemption. In this, a majority of Indian cancer memoirs resemble many of their global counterparts that similarly promise identification and consolation to their readers, without necessarily acknowledging the preconditions of these promises. This global cohort of cancer memoirs elides the structural and collective barriers that hinder survival; for instance, they say very little about the difficulties for those without means to access timely treatments, or about the fact that only a subset of cancers are amenable to therapies that lead to long-term remission.

At the same time as I explained my dissatisfaction with these dominant tendencies of cancer memoirs, in this chapter I have also described three that went against their generic grain. These placed the crisis of the disease within longer histories of vulnerability, connecting the precarity of lives before and after diagnosis. I found that these three memoirs provided an "emic" account of what it meant to live and die with cancer, in a way that was consistent with my ethnographic descriptions. *My Mother Did Not Go Bald* trafficked in the same complexity of concealment and the possibilities of subjunctive life I found in my work with Cansupport. The choreography of telling and not telling allowed for multiple, even contradictory, modes of living with and alongside cancer—concretized in the memoir's form as a list of thirty-two bystanders. Formal composition joined narrative storytelling to capture what is a key insight of my book, too: that cancer fragments life into many "as-ifs," which become crucial modes through which the disease folds into everyday life. Similarly, *Mayan* was a commentary on possibilities of violence and recognition that are opened in the wake of a cancer diagnosis. Like many physicians and kin who have appeared in my ethnographic accounts, Vineet sought to understand his mother's pain and suffering, even in the face of the vast gulf that separated their experiences of the disease. But, as well-intentioned as his desires to empathize were, they forced a second violence on Mayan, the violence of his misrecognition as he overwhelmed her experience with his own imagination of what an ethical and good death should look like. In this, his efforts resembled those of some of the cancer pain researchers I described in the previous chapter, who similarly sought to empathize and offer pathways to transcendence through a recourse to mythic figures. But while those physicians never rejected analgesia, Vineet's desire to transcend his mother's pain was so complete that he urged her to do so, achieving a more authentic, painful death. In this way, the sevā Vineet offered to Mayan mingled violence and care, even though he did not recognize it as doing so. Finally, the gendered dimensions of misrecognition were similarly replete in *Silent Echoes*. For Prerna, cancer appeared as a postscript to a long history of domestic and affinal violence. Explicitly, she refused to draw clear lines between the violence of her social world and that of her disease, choosing instead to trace the lines of care and violence that ran through both.

In the next chapter, I turn to film and continue to ask the following questions of aesthetic accounts of cancer: How do they narrativize the doubts and skepticisms about the self and social relations in the shadow of cancer? And how do they imagine recovery in the face of such doubts? In these memoirs, we have seen two contrasting answers to these questions. For some accounts, cancer became a mode of chastisement, a lesson to correct past shortcomings and failures in the search for a better life after the disease. Such a mode of representing cancer presumed its pedagogical capacity to reform social worlds. But in another set of accounts, cancer offered no easy path to redemption. Rather, these accounts presented a patient's vulnerability to cancer not as a somaticized outcome of past sins or lifestyle choices but as biological duress coupled with a durative fragility in relations that preceded and outlived the disease. For such accounts, restitution and resolution were not easy, even if they were a desired horizon. These accounts come closest to my ethnographic description of the social—as a network of fragile relations whose capacities for strength and support are tested by a cancer diagnosis. They supplement my ethnographic efforts to show how any effort to ameliorate cancer requires working within and through the fragile social ties within which the disease often takes shape.

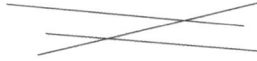

5

CANCER FILMS

Medical practitioners in India often complain that Indian films about cancer present a disheartening picture of the disease to patients. In 2015, a well-known public health specialist—Sanghamitra Pati—took to the *Lancet* to diagnose the Indian film industry as itself cancerous.[1] Pati expressed disappointment that cancer patients in Indian films always died. Instead of depicting cancer "realistically," she argued, Indian filmmakers were "misleading" people about cancer by concealing the possibility of recovery. Her concern was that this "cancerous" industry was spreading its fear to those "without health literacy in rural and urban areas," whom she believed to be popular cinema's primary audience. She then went further to say that filmmakers had fallen out of step with national progress regarding early diagnosis and innovative treatments. Other public health experts have expressed the same concerns about Hindi films about cancer in journals and at conferences.[2] And this disapprobation is not confined to specialist discussions; it also appears in patients' own accounts. For example, in a collection of short accounts collated by an oncologist at a private hospital in Delhi, a patient recalls that his first thought after receiving his diagnosis was about Indian cancer films and how "they install fear in the hearts of thousands of cancer patients and thousands of families of cancer patients."[3]

Indian films about cancer are certainly suffused with pathos, and their critics are not wrong in pointing out an absence of narratives in which patients recover and survive the diagnosis. Yet, I caution against the deceptively self-evident claims that pathos misrepresents experiences of the disease and hinders the well-being of patients. Scholars of Indian cinema have long warned against such elite disdain of Indian popular culture and those who consume it. Ravi Vasudevan, for example, describes how the aesthetics of popular cinema are devalued by highbrow filmmakers and critics, while Tejaswini Ganti finds that even contemporary filmmakers are often disdainful of their audiences.[4] Moving past elite suspicions, I suggest here that Indian films provide some of the most complex accounts of what it means to live with cancer. Further, I find these cinematic depictions compelling for the same reason they trouble doctors and public health specialists—their embrace of pathos. If the generic cancer memoir described in the previous chapter promises a fantasy of assured recovery and survivorship, Indian films refuse this consolation. Instead, they stay with the trouble cancer produces in social relations.

Films about cancer thus extend my ethnographic work as culturally emic, metasocial commentaries that stand as interpretive texts alongside my own. I think of them not as offering new empirical cases but as offering contrasting conceptual frames that help develop my analysis of the face-to-face ethnographic work. These films share many of the concerns that run through my ethnography—explicitly thematizing sacrifices demanded in the disease's wake, concealments as forms of care, the violence of misrecognition, and the desire to transcend suffering. At the same time, in their persistent desire to dramatize and resolve these themes on a broad cultural-historical canvas, they depart from the irresolute and proximal registers of my ethnography. In what follows, I trace this tension between my proximal ethnographic work and the more ambitious distal registers of Indian cancer films.

Healing the Nation

Released in 1963, *Dil Ek Mandir* was the first in a succession of films about cancer that are now canonical in postcolonial Hindi cinema.[5] It starred three of the most well-known actors of the time—Rajendra Kumar, Meena Kumari, and Raj Kumar as Ram, Sita, and Dharmesh. The names of the films' protagonists invoke the Ramayana, an epic that has generated countless retellings across Asia for more than three millennia. The myth centers on the young Prince Ram and his wife, Sita. Early in the epic, the couple are exiled from their kingdom by the machinations of Ram's stepmother. During their exile, Sita is abducted by the Lankan demon-king Ravana. Ram assembles an army, kills Ravana, and rescues Sita. Ram then demands proof that Sita

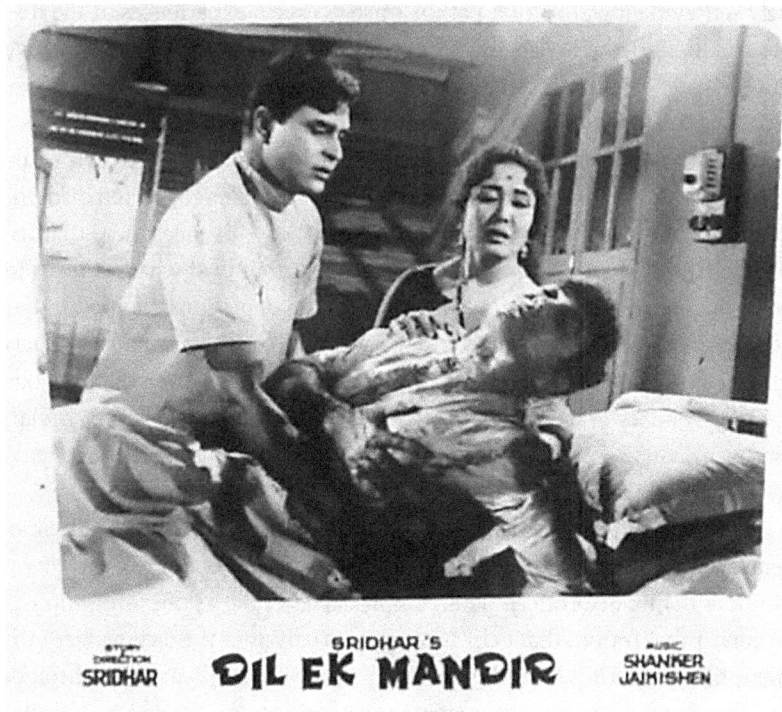

FIGURE 5.1 Lobby card for *Dil Ek Mandir* (1963). Photo from Osianama Research Centre Archive, Library and Sanctuary, India.

remained faithful and chaste during her abduction, and so she enters a fire to prove her fidelity. Ram accepts her back after she emerges unharmed, and they both return to their kingdom at the end of their exile. The period of Ram's rule following his restitution inaugurates Ram Rajya—a mythic kingdom and age of peace and prosperity. Crucially for its narrative, *Dil Ek Mandir* aligns itself with this mythic story by naming its main protagonists Ram and Sita.

The film begins with a present-day Ram and Sita coming to Dharmesh for medical care. Ram is a wealthy young man who has been diagnosed with cancer, and Dharmesh is a renowned cancer surgeon. A series of flash-backs reveals that Sita and Dharmesh were lovers before she married Ram. The film unfolds in Dharmesh's cancer hospital and around this tense re-lational triangle. Early in the film, Ram discovers Sita and Dharmesh's past relationship and follows her to see if their love has been rekindled. The invocation here is unmistakably that of Ram testing Sita's chastity in the

Ramayana. If mythic Sita turns out to be beyond reproach, so does filmic Sita. If anything, she is troubled that her past romantic entanglement with Dharmesh might interfere with his present medical duty to save Ram. But Dharmesh is no Ravana. (While his name is not a referent to the Ramayana, it translates as "master of righteousness.") If the epic pits Ram against Ravana and thus good against evil, the contest in the film is between Ram and Dharmesh—two paragons of ethical virtue. Ram spends the days leading up to his surgery trying to convince Dharmesh to marry Sita in the event of the surgery's failure. He does this not only hoping to ensure Sita's future happiness but also expressing his desire to take part in the reformist, postcolonial social project of widow remarriage.[6] Dharmesh refuses him this promise. Instead, he responds by redoubling his commitment to his medical vocation and is consumed by his desire to save Ram. A montage shows him refusing food or sleep, while he agonizes over the procedure and pores over the latest research and protocols. He drives himself to exhaustion and dies moments after successfully performing the surgery, but not before he staggers to a waiting Sita to tell her that Ram will live (figure 5.2). The final scene of the film sanctifies Dharmesh's sacrifice: the couple inaugurate a philanthropic hospital and dedicate it to Dharmesh's memory (figure 5.3).

As Wendy Doniger writes, many versions of the Ramayana elevate Ram and Sita as exemplars of moral virtue.[7] Such versions have proved popular with the contemporary religious right in India, which purports to re-create Ram's mythic (read Hindu) kingdom in the present. Released in 1963, however, *Dil Ek Mandir* narrativizes a different political vision. The film invokes the Ramayana not to articulate an exclusionary nativism but to commemorate the hope that science and medicine held for many of the postcolonial Indian elite as a panacea to the nation's problems. At one level, the film is a straightforward allegory for the sacrifices demanded by the new nation-state, with scientists and doctors as the exemplary figures capable of selflessness. Cancer becomes an opportunity to demonstrate selfless sacrifice for the nation-state, embodied in the figure of the chaste Indian woman.

However, such a straightforward reading obscures filmic Sita's claims to recognition. She is more than just a mute figure over which male paragons stake their moral contest. Consider her journey through the film's narrative. Through the first half of the film, Dharmesh's mother and Ram malign the moral laxity of that unnamed woman in Dharmesh's past who betrayed him. They do not know that the object of their condemnation is really Sita, who remains silent under the burden of these accusations. In public, Dharmesh defends this woman in his past, elevating her to the status of a goddess equal

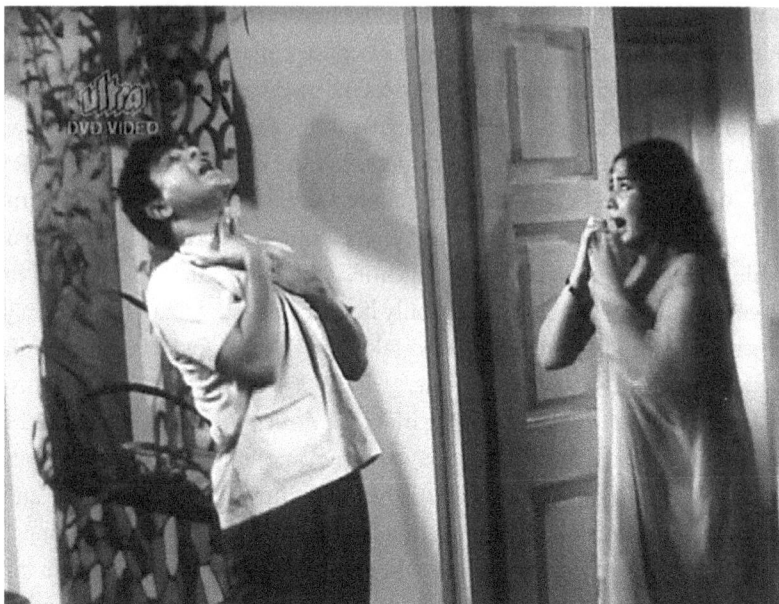

FIGURE 5.2 Still from *Dil Ek Mandir* (1963). Dharmesh dies at the moment of telling Sita that Ram will be cured.

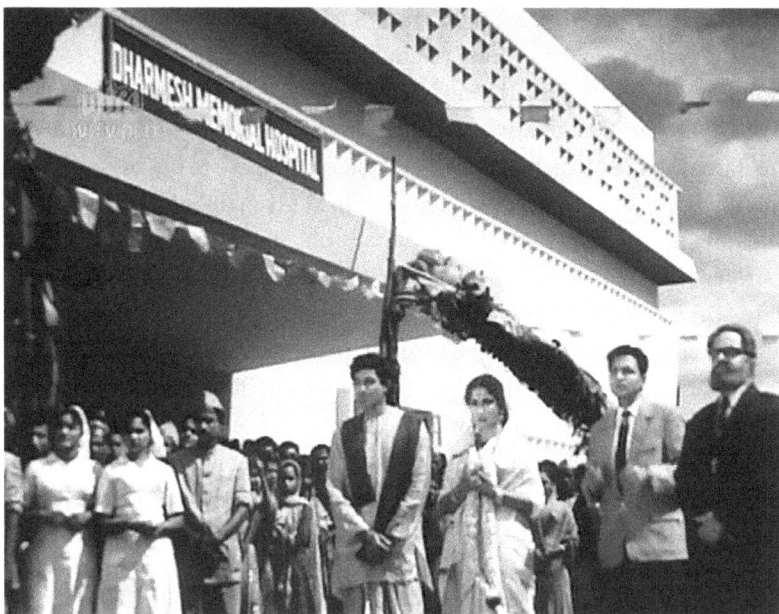

FIGURE 5.3 Still from *Dil Ek Mandir* (1963). Ram and Sita commemorate Dharmesh by building a charitable hospital in his memory.

to his vocation. But while speaking privately to Sita, Dharmesh joins with these accusations, questioning her decision to leave him. Sita breaks her silence at this critical moment. She reveals that her father had been in debt to Ram's father, who had agreed to forgive the debt if Sita married Ram. At the time, Ram had not been told of his diagnosis. Thus, while the protagonists of the film accuse Sita of betrayal, she reveals instead the more difficult moral choice that had been put before her—the choice between familial dishonor and personal love. In contrast to the moral clarity of Dharmesh's and Ram's self-sacrifice, then, we find Sita navigating a much trickier ethical terrain, where neither choice before her allows for virtuous resolution. As the narrative unfolds, Sita comes to embody the weight of her ethical burden, fainting in a hysterical fit as the camera dances at acute angles to capture her derangement (figure 5.5). In moments such as these in the film, Sita's derangement allows us a glimpse into the elisions and violence in Ram's and Dharmesh's quest for martyrdom made possible through their relation to cancer.

Dil Ek Mandir set into place a recognizable trope for Indian films about cancer in the 1960s: the disease interrupts the lives of cinematic protagonists and demands from them sacrifices to a national cause. In these films, cancer affords protagonists a chance to seize the disease as an opportunity to transcend their immediate difficulties, giving up their lives for the sake of the newly decolonized nation. But while the explicit sacrifice is often gendered male, the sacrifice of women is more subtly coded. They often bear the durative burden of the consequences of these heroic martyrdoms, living on with the knowledge of the sacrifice made on their behalf, while being disallowed the opportunity or voice to make the same sacrifices. C. V. Sridhar—who directed *Dil Ek Mandir*—made another cancer film in 1968 that further entrenched this trope.

Saathi begins with Ravi—a brilliant oncologist—returning from the United States to aid the Indian poor. He falls in love with Shanti, a nurse at the hospital where he works. Shanti and Ravi become close when her mother is diagnosed with cancer. When Shanti's mother dies, Shanti and Ravi commit themselves to marriage, driven not only by love but also by their commitment to serving the nation by finding a cure for cancer together. But while Ravi's research flourishes, Shanti develops a heart condition she hides from him. In the film's first sacrifice, Shanti runs away so that she no longer distracts him from his vocation. Soon after, Ravi receives news that Shanti has died. Ravi is distraught and devotes himself to his work. He agrees to remarry out of respect for his stepparents, who have always wanted him to marry their daughter Rajni. Rajni tries to take Shanti's place in his life, but

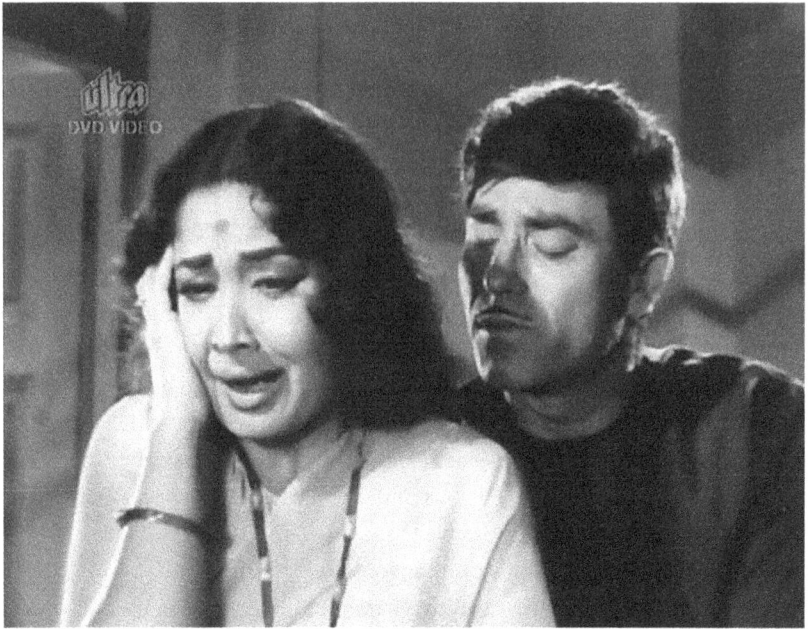

FIGURE 5.4 Still from *Dil Ek Mandir* (1963). Ram asks Sita to reconcile with his death.

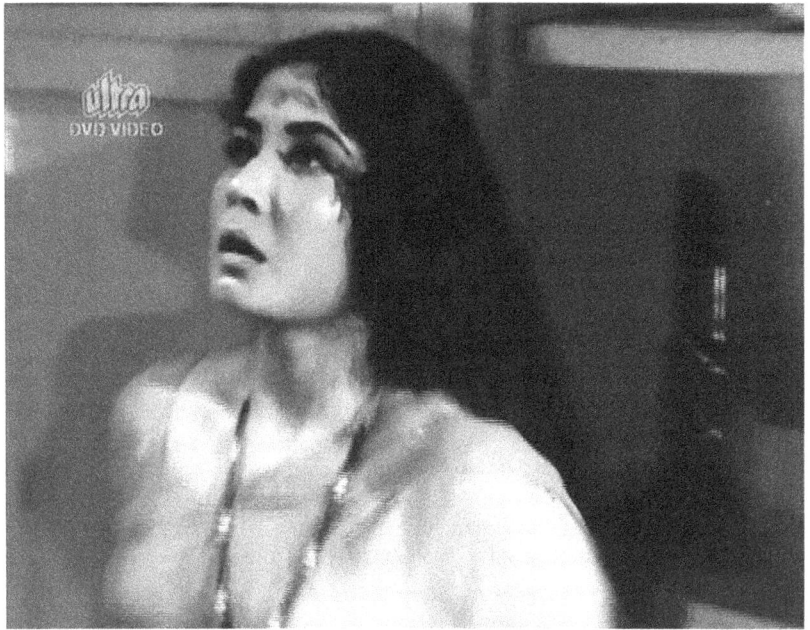

FIGURE 5.5 Still from *Dil Ek Mandir* (1963). Sita is about to collapse under the weight of her sacrifice.

he insists that she does not show the same ethical high-mindedness. Driven to despair by Ravi's inattention, Rajni tries to commit suicide by drinking the chemicals in his laboratory. Ravi intervenes to save her but is blinded in the process.

In a maneuver typical of the Indian melodrama, an unlikely coincidence leads to an unexpected revelation: we find that Shanti is not only alive but also cured of her heart ailment. She returns to Ravi but, finding him married to Rajni, resolves to conceal her identity. Instead, she enacts another sacrifice—she assumes a different name and nurses Ravi, aiming to return him to cancer research. Ravi, however, is distracted; grieving for Shanti, he refuses surgery. He talks of his love for Shanti (whom he still presumes dead) as a mirror of Ram's love for Sita in the Ramayana. However, with much effort, Shanti coaxes him to agree to the surgery. Her duty fulfilled, she then seeks to enact a third sacrifice by killing herself for the sake of Ravi's marriage. But with his sight restored, Ravi saves Shanti just in time, finally recognizing her to be his dead wife come back to life. These exemplary sacrifices are too much for Rajni, who bears witness to Ravi and Shanti's unerring commitment to cancer research. Inspired by Shanti's selflessness, she abandons her attachment to Ravi and commits herself to becoming a nurse, allowing Shanti and Ravi to reunite in marriage. If *Dil Ek Mandir* established the cancer film as a canvas for male self-sacrifice to the vocation of medicine, *Saathi* allows for female sacrifices for similarly lofty goals. At the same time, the echoes of *Dil Ek Mandir* are unmistakable; *Saathi* reiterates its message that conjugal and romantic love must be sacrificed for a greater cause—finding a treatment and cure for cancer, which in turn demonstrates the ideological ambitions of postcolonial India and its newly inspired citizens.

The sanctity of the newly decolonized nation in *Dil Ek Mandir* and *Saathi* frames the sacrifices it demands as both necessary and self-evident. But *Satyakam*, released a year after *Saathi* in 1968, presents a more cynical view of the postcolonial nation-state. The film's narrative begins in the year of Indian independence. The protagonists, a cohort of engineering students, feel all the optimism of the promise of decolonization. The film follows two of these students, Satyapriya and his friend Narendra, both of whom look forward to a life of nation-building, service, and social renewal. Soon, however, Satyapriya's life falls apart. His name translates to "a love of truth," and it is precisely his uncompromising fidelity that is his downfall. Even as he seeks to build the infrastructure of a new nation with dams and bridges, he is confronted by the persistence of feudal corruption that has seeped into the national bureaucracy. Satyapriya refuses to make the moral concessions

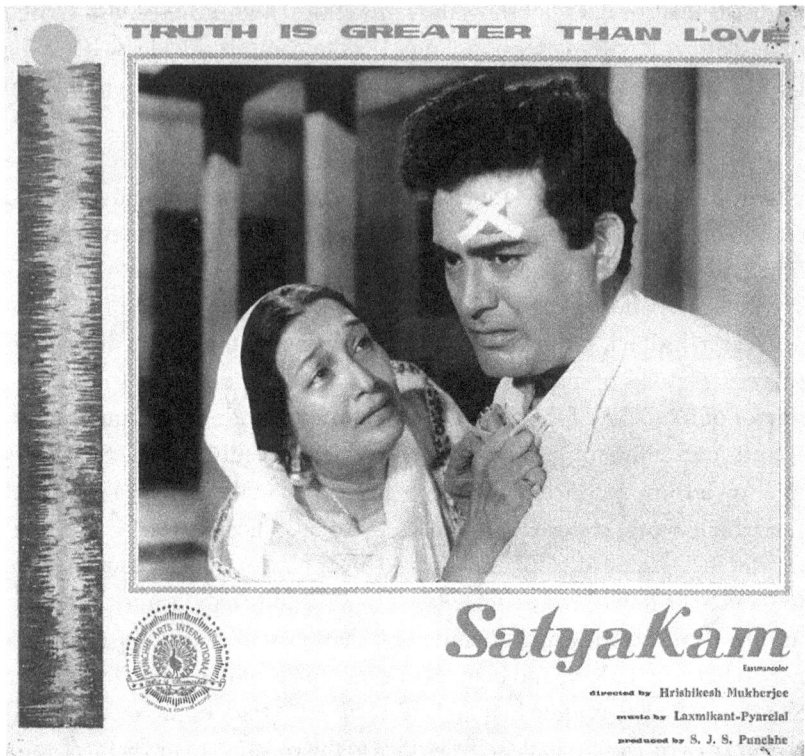

FIGURE 5.6 Still mounted on lobby card for *Satyakam* (1969). Image from Osianama Research Centre Archive, Library and Sanctuary, India.

demanded of him, and he is fired from one job after another. He is forced to abandon his engineering dreams, resigning himself to working as a poorly paid state regulator. In the meantime, he marries Ranjana—a dancer whose reputation is left in question after she is assaulted by a feudal lord. Even as he partially repairs her social standing through marriage, Satyapriya loses his own and finds himself isolated from his kin.

Finally, Satyapriya is diagnosed with lung cancer, brought about by his one and only vice: the cigarettes he smokes to ameliorate the stress of the poverty brought on by his high moral code. It is as if the failed promise of the Indian nation-state brings about Satyapriya's disease. After his cancer diagnosis, Satyapriya's condition quickly deteriorates, and his wife faces a difficult moral choice. Through the course of the film, Ranjana is devoted to him, even as his moral code leaves them in poverty. As Satyapriya lies on his deathbed, Ranjana despairs over how she and their child will survive after his death. At this moment, a man from Satyapriya's past approaches her with a plan, promising Ranjana money and future security if she can convince Satyapriya to approve a dubious engineering project. By this time, Satyapriya's cancer has progressed so far that he cannot speak. When Ranjana comes to him with the papers that might ensure her future, he looks disappointed but nevertheless signs them, breaking for the first time in his life from his moral code. While taking the papers from him, Ranjana sees the sadness in Satyapriya's eyes and rips them up. As his final act of authority in the film, Satyapriya smiles approvingly. At the precise moment he loses his voice, Ranjana becomes a cipher for his moral certitude, while taking on the burden of its unrelenting violence into her future.

Satyakam forms a triad of 1960s cancer films with *Dil Ek Mandir* and *Saathi*. In each, the conjuncture of cancer, kinship, and nation compels sacrifices from its protagonists. It is not accidental that all three films share the generic form of the melodrama—a popular aesthetic that runs through Hindi cinema, with especially particular intensity in the 1950s and 1960s. As it happens, the choice of melodrama as a generic mode was a felicitous one in representing cancer. The genre, often castigated by critics for departing from the ideal of realism, offered several opportunities for thematizing the trope of sacrifice that is at the center of these films. Definitionally, melodramas portray virtuous protagonists beset by forces more powerful than they are, enacting a pathos of suffering in response to powerlessness.[8] In these films, cancer stands in for the tragedy that has overwhelmed virtuous protagonists, depriving them of control over their lives and actions. But, as is typical with melodramas, these films framed the violence of the disease within a much more encompassing canvas than personal despair. Indeed, the felicity of the form is how it connects vastly disparate scales—the personal, the familial, and the national—allowing them to imagine the reverberations of a cancer diagnosis across the disparate domains. In Peter Brooks's canonical description of the melodrama, the mode emerges in the wake of modern social and political transformations, focusing narrative attention on the disjointed interior states of its protagonists.[9] More specifically, melodramas seize upon the perceived disjunction in these times of how things are and how they should be, and how this disjunction impinges on their protagonists' quest for fulfillment. In Hindi films of the time, the social disjunction was between the promise of decolonization and a reality of the social inequalities that persisted in its wake. For *Dil Ek Mandir* and *Saathi*, still animated by decolonial hope and promise, male protagonists seized upon cancer as a mode through which to enact social reform through personal sacrifice. But if Dharmesh's death in *Dil Ek Mandir* still took part in the heady potentiality of national reform, Satyapriya's death in *Satyakam* revealed decolonization's disappointment. Reform through sacrifice was no longer a possibility. Through the melodramatic form, then, these early films achieve a magnification of cancer onto a national scale. The form of the melodrama opened the personal to the national and the private to the public in ways that offered a fascinating commentary on the disease.

The Magical Cancer Patient

Importantly, Ravi Vasudevan qualifies Brooks's description of the melodrama to show how its Indian iteration privileged not individual interiority but that of the family.[10] The sacrifice of men thus takes place not only in relation to the nation but also in relation to the men's familial roles, alongside the subtler disjunction between the interior and public lives of their wives. That is, while protagonists could often seize control of their fates by enacting a will to martyrdom, the sacrifice of women was far more subtly coded. If Ram, Dharmesh, Ravi, and Satyapriya each dictated the form and orientation of their sacrifice, women in the films bore the consequences of their moral choices, compelled to witness and make sacrifices not always of their choosing. In *Dil Ek Mandir*, Sita bore the poisonous past of having been sold to Ram for the sake of familial honor. In *Saathi*, Shanti denied herself happiness to the point of self-destruction, so that Ravi's sacrifices might be writ large upon the nation. And, most tellingly, in *Satyakam*, Ranjana and her child were sentenced to a lifetime of poverty, but only after she learned to choose this suffering for herself at Satyapriya's deathbed. The pathos of women in these melodramas was never a resolved concern (as it was for men who earned salvation through sacrifice) but an essential blockage that could not be transcended. Women's suffering was durative in a way that condemned them to an enduring abjection.

For feminist film critics studying this kind of representation of women in melodrama, this tendency of the genre to dramatize abject female suffering without resolution posed a problem.[11] These critics were uncomfortable with the denial of agency and the passivity in these portrayals while they sought at the same time to recuperate the power of melodramatic pathos. Christine Gledhill presented a way out of this bind by suggesting that the root of melodramatic pathos was not simply the spectacle of suffering but the revelation of the violence of recognition.[12] That is, Gledhill argued that the pathos of melodrama was because audiences—made aware of a "true" context—

became witnesses to a universe in which the actions of female protagonists were fated to misrecognition. This is a persuasive way to read the representations of Sita, Shanti, and Ranjana. Their suffering testifies not to their passive victimhood but to the structure of recognition in which only certain kinds of martyrdom (gendered male) can find fulfillment. Their sacrifices—to bear the durative burden of male sacrifices on their behalf but not of their choosing—are not allowed to become the central structuring principle of the film. But in certain moments I described, their sacrifices erupt onto the filmic screen. For brief moments, women externalized their previously unexpressed interior selves, partially through words, but also through action.[13] Most evocatively, this eruption appeared in Sita's near-hysterical collapse, as she captured in gesture and movement the structure of misrecognition in which she was consistently denied voice. More subtly, it appeared as Rajni's will to self-harm, driven to desperation by her violent rejection by Ravi, who is literally blinded by his desire to sacrifice himself to find a cure. And it appeared also in Shanti's and Sita's near deaths, as they bore the violence of misrecognition in which their sacrifices could find no words, while those of their husbands turned them into heroic martyrs to the cause of cancer's cure.

If Indian films about cancer in the 1960s represented the gendered relation between nation, disease, and sacrifice, the next decade witnessed a dramatic change in this cinematic orientation. Even as *Satyakam* became a critical success in later decades, the film's contemporaneous commercial failure prompted its director, Hrishikesh Mukherjee, to doubt the pedagogical capacity of cinema to educate and incite social change.[14] His next film grew out of this disappointment and resulted in the most well-known cultural representation of cancer in India. Released in 1971, *Anand* tells the story of a cancer patient living out his last months with the disease. In contrast to *Satyakam*, the film received immediate critical and commercial acclaim and launched the career of Indian cinema's most famous actor, Amitabh Bachchan. *Anand* begins where *Satyakam* leaves off: Bachchan plays Bhaskar Banerjee, a doctor driven to alcoholism by the failure of the promise of decolonization. The first shots of the film include a montage of destitution in urban slums, as Bhaskar wanders around in frustration, unable to ease the suffering of the urban poor.

Recall that in *Satyakam* cancer appears as an outcome of Satyapriya's unwavering moral code, allowing him to demonstrate his incorruptibility even in the face of death. Class is front and center in that film's narrative. Satyapriya is driven to destitution, while his more corrupt counterparts thrive; the difference between him and the social world he lives in narrativizes the

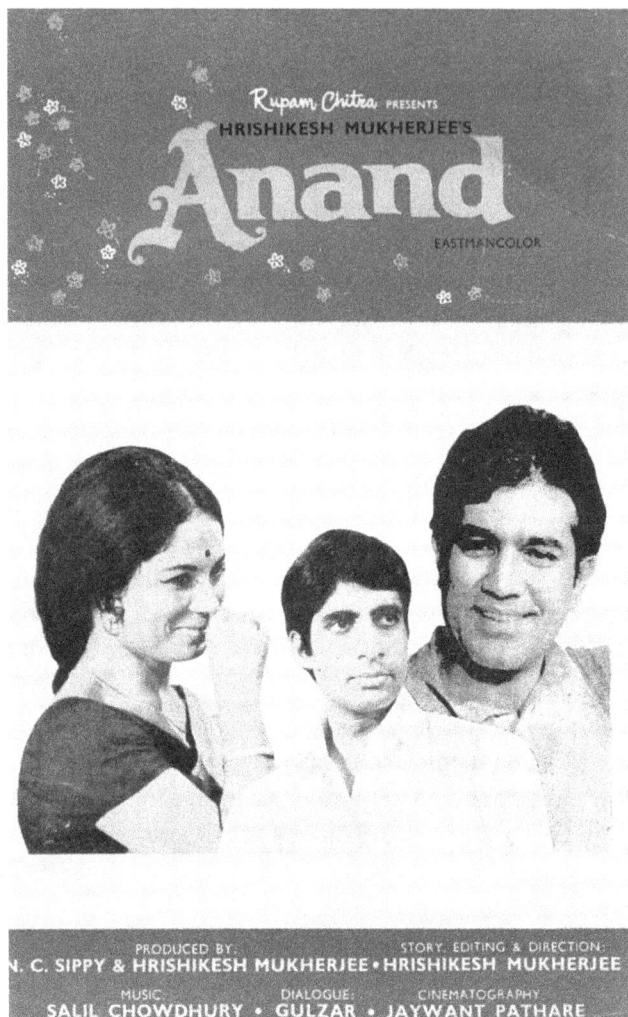

FIGURE 5.7 Song synopsis booklet for *Anand* (1971). Image from Osianama Research Centre Archive, Library and Sanctuary, India.

abject failure of the promise of decolonization. In *Anand*, cancer fulfills a remarkably different narrative function: it helps evade difficult moral choices. Bhaskar is rescued from his despondency about social inequality by Anand's relentless cheerfulness.[15] Anand confounds Bhaskar and compels his undivided attention because he seems magically unaffected by his terminal prognosis; he makes no demands of treatment or sacrifice. If Anand is exemplary, his example demonstrates that by turning away from difficult social questions, happiness remains available to those who are able to seize it through personal will. Thus, Anand sings and laughs his way through the film, while politely recusing himself from company at the first sign of physi-

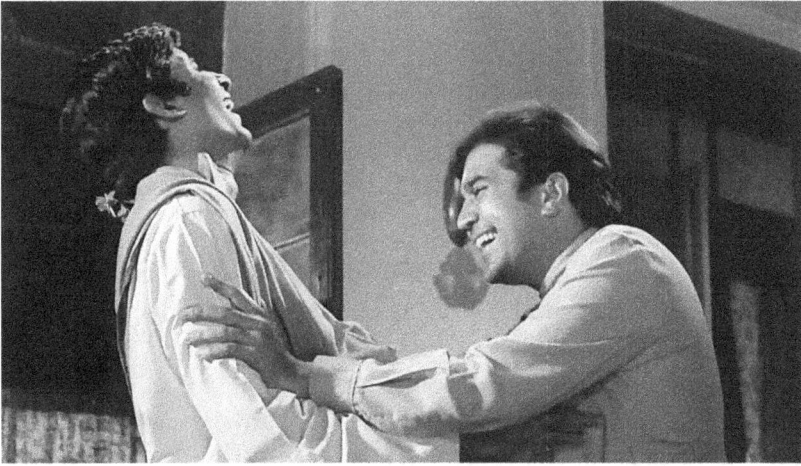

FIGURE 5.8 Still from *Anand* (1971). Anand lifts Dr. Banerjee's spirits, moments before his final collapse.

cal symptoms, coughing up blood in privacy. Lawrence Cohen describes this humanism of Anand as perverse: despite Bhaskar's early anger at state failure, the film suggests that death comes as inexorably even to the middle class, in the shape of cancer.[16] It is no longer class that matters in determining disease and death, then, but the ability of patients and kin to bear suffering with resilience and optimism.

Bolstered by *Anand's* success, Hrishikesh Mukherjee made another cancer film soon afterward. Released in 1974, *Milli* told the story of a female cancer patient whom many critics describe as a female version of Anand. As with *Anand*, the title of the film is eponymous with its protagonist, who responds to her diagnosis with a frightening degree of cheerfulness and hyperactivity. As with *Anand*, the role of every supporting character in *Milli* is to marvel at her spirit. And as with *Anand*, the despairing character played by Amitabh Bachchan is the foil to Milli's optimism. *Milli* unfolds much in the same way as *Anand*; over the course of the film, Milli transforms Bachchan's despair into love and optimism. At the end of their respective films, Anand dies and Milli's death looms. But through their deaths, they offer restitution and recovery to proximate others, rescuing them from anomie and despair. Even as they cannot recover from their own illnesses, Milli and Anand return life to others.

In one respect, then, *Anand* and *Milli* resembled the Indian cancer films that preceded them in that the disease is transformative of all those who encounter it. But if transformation in the 1960s meant selfless sacrifices to the nation, the telos of change is much less ambitious in the films of the early 1970s. The orientation of sacrifice is not toward a nation but, more modestly, toward palliating the psychological distress of proximate friends, families, or lovers.

Dramas of Disclosure

Hindi cancer films that followed *Anand* and *Milli* continued to focus on the distress suffered by those surrounding the one who is ill, but they did so without the magical cancer patient as their primary narrative agent. Rather, the dramatic events in this next set of films were motivated by crises brought on by the concealment and disclosure of the cancer diagnosis. These films are a fascinating analogue to the cancer concealment described in prior chapters, where I found my fieldwork interlocutors exploring the possibilities of the subjunctive—of living in the space of the "as-if"—offered by partial and strategic concealments. The protagonists of films about concealment resemble my ethnographic interlocutors in that they too traffic in the indeterminacies of partial disclosures. At the same time, the narrative structures of these films force moments of dramatic reckoning and confession that were often deftly avoided by my interlocutors in my face-to-face fieldwork. In this, the films offer up a contrastive mirror to my ethnography, dramatizing the stakes of disclosure.

To elaborate, these films of the late 1970s and 1980s portrayed disclosure as an event as devastating and dramatic as the diagnosis. Released in 1978, *Ankhiyon Ke Jharokhon Se* (The window of the eyes) provides a good example. The film centers on the love between two undergraduate students, Sachin and Lily. When Lily falls unwell, she is taken by her mother to a doctor for diagnosis. The film then tracks a cascading series of concealments and disclosures. First, the doctor who receives her tests hesitates to tell Lily's mother. When he finally does, the film cuts to an explosive hiss from a pressure-release valve in the doctor's laboratory; the sound drowns out the utterance of the word "cancer" and the mother's subsequent scream and collapse. This filmic metaphor describes the subsequent series of disclosures: each unblocks and releases pent-up narrative tension. Lily's mother hides the diagnosis from Lily, who only finds out she has cancer after spying on both her mother and the doctor. This is the first time the film allows the word "cancer" to be spoken. Lily then pretends to her mother she does not know, hoping to spare her a difficult conversation, instead presenting a hyperactive

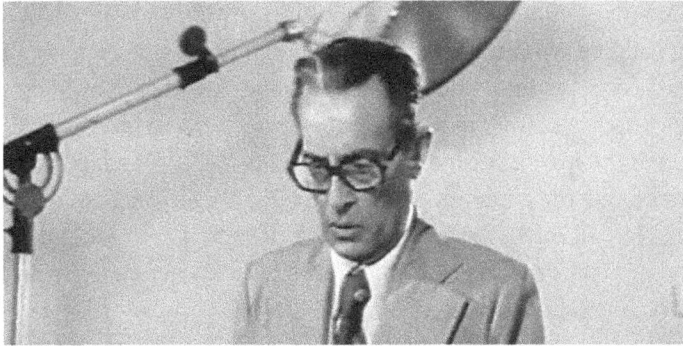

FIGURE 5.9 Still from *Ankhiyon Ke Jharokhon Se* (1978). The doctor hesitates to tell the diagnosis.

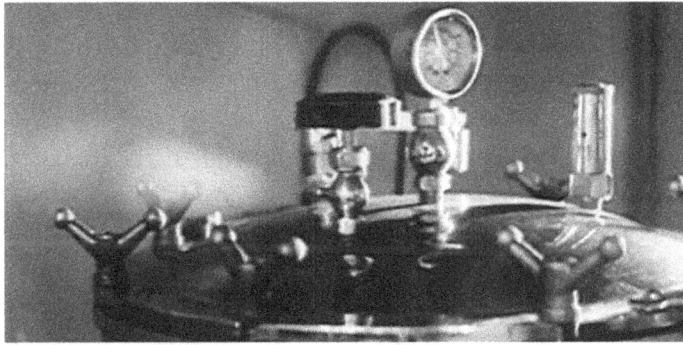

FIGURE 5.10 Still from *Ankhiyon Ke Jharokhon Se* (1978). The film cuts to the hiss of a scientific pressure machine releasing steam and drowning out the word "cancer."

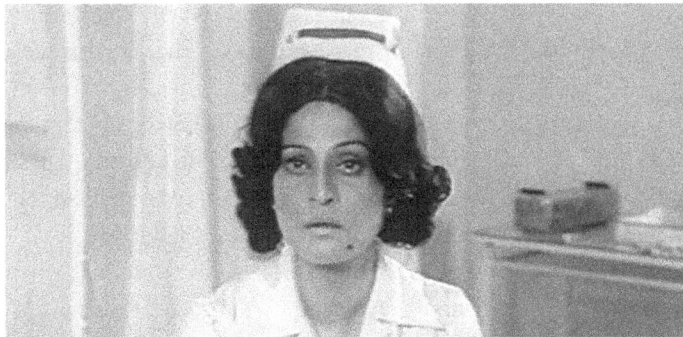

FIGURE 5.11 Still from *Ankhiyon Ke Jharokhon Se* (1978). Lily's mother is left in catatonic shock after hearing the word "cancer."

cheerfulness to disguise her own shock. But unlike in *Milli* and *Anand*, this cheerfulness collapses within minutes; Lily cannot keep up the pretense of optimism and collapses into a deep catatonic shock. At this point, Lily's mother goes to Sachin's father to break off the couple's engagement. Again, she tries to hide the reason behind her decision. She collapses again when Sachin's father forces the truth out of her, as if felled by the weight of uttering the word. Now all three conspire to hide the diagnosis from Sachin. He is understandably confused and only finds out the truth when he overhears his father talking to Lily's doctor.

For a brief period in the film, everybody knows Lily has cancer, and they all hope and fight for her treatment. The faith of the 1960s films in the Indian medical vocation is absent in this film; instead, the characters wait desperately for an American cancer doctor to arrive and cure Lily. Lily, however, does not live long enough for this foreign operation.[17] The film ends with Sachin becoming a doctor, promising to live on, inspired by Lily's sacrifice. Sachin's elegiac commitment to his vocation echoes the centrality of sacrifice in early Indian cancer films. But the echo is faint, and sacrifice is an afterthought to a narrative preoccupation with disclosure. Thus, cancer's function as a narrative device shifts again. Sacrifice to another—nation, friend, or lover—remains a central preoccupation. At the same time, sacrifice takes the form of concealing the diagnosis. In other words, the burden of sacrifice spreads across kinship relations, demanding that each protagonist show his or her capacity for selflessness by taking turns in swallowing and hiding the poisonous knowledge of cancer.

Released in 1981, *Prem Geet* (Love song) raises these new narrative stakes of concealment and disclosure. The film follows the love between a poet and a dancer—Akash and Shikha. When Shikha becomes ill, Akash takes her to a doctor, who cryptically tells Akash to break off his engagement with Shikha. When pressed, the doctor reveals to Akash that Shikha has a brain tumor. Both Akash and the doctor conspire to hide the diagnosis from Shikha. Akash goes on to marry Shikha despite knowing her terminal prognosis, hoping to give her a few months of happiness before her death. At first, Akash's father is opposed to the marriage, but he comes around when told of Shikha's diagnosis and the high-mindedness of Akash's sacrifice. Akash and his father now resolve to keep the diagnosis from Akash's mother. Much of the film unfolds as a drama where the male protagonists bear the poisonous knowledge of Shikha's cancer, while the female protagonists—Shikha and Akash's mother—celebrate an imminent marriage. After marriage, as Shikha's condition deteriorates, Akash allows both women to believe that

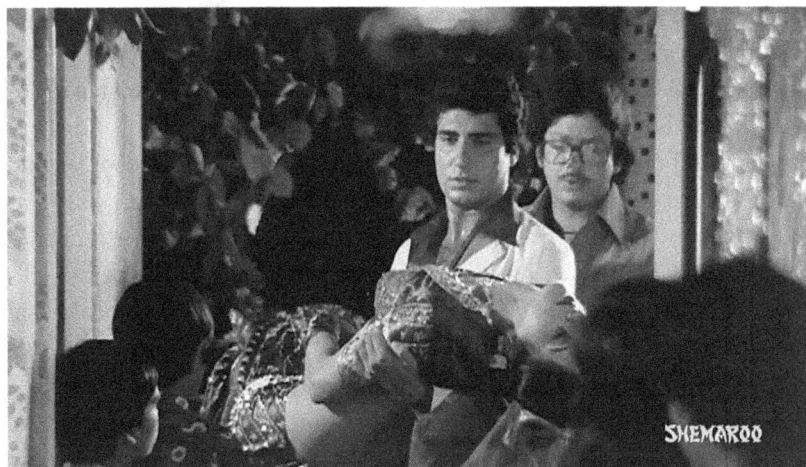

FIGURE 5.12 Still from *Prem Geet* (1981). Akash carries Shikha back across the threshold of his house moments before her death.

her physical symptoms are symptoms of a pregnancy. As the family prepares for a fictitious child, Akash's sacrifice takes on more serious proportions. Eventually, Shikha finds out about her own diagnosis during a visit to a gynecologist. Determined to outdo Akash's sacrifice and to return his gift of concealment, she convinces her doctor not to let anyone else know that she knows. Her final gesture in the film is to perform a last dance at a benefit for a cancer hospital. Akash finds her and stops her before she begins her performance. It is as if the privilege of sacrifice is the provenance of only the male protagonists in the film. Shikha dies moments after Akash's rescue, as he carries her dying body back into the threshold of the domestic.

With *Prem Geet*, we have come a long way from the early cancer films, even as it shares their trope of sacrifice. Even as women appeared as stereotypes of self-abnegation in those early films, they retained a capacity for knowledge and action. Sita, Shanti, and Ranjana wielded their knowledge and their agentive capability to sacrifice, even as their knowledge and sacrifice were misrecognized and eclipsed by their male counterparts. But Akash denies Shikha even the gesture of a muted self-sacrifice. Not only is she kept from the knowledge of her disease, but the other characters also lead her to believe she is pregnant. Confined to inactivity and domesticity, she is rendered incapable of speech or action to give her own death meaning.

In Peter Brooks's canonical description of the form, the power of melodrama is its ability to put forward in gesture, music, or pantomime what cannot be put forward in words. As such, the melodramatic form offers powerful possibilities in representing a disease whose experience and representation are replete with elisions and concealments. But here, the enactment of melodrama takes on a different affective telos. In the films of the 1960s and 1970s, the genre afforded women the possibility to testify—through embodied and gestural excess—to the structure of misrecognition in which their voice was fated to never be heard. In these later films, the subject of sacrifice is no longer the nation or a greater social good, but the immediate psychological well-being of the woman herself. Women no longer stand in for projects of social reform but become voiceless, passive sufferers. They can no longer even sacrifice themselves for a greater social good. Rather than opening spaces and possibilities of expression, these films further constrain the range of women's expressiveness. The performative excess of Shikha's desire to dance and turn her cancer into a charity benefit is halted because it threatens to eclipse her husband's sacrifice for her. In these dramas of disclosure, women are no longer active helpers in transforming cancer into a reformist national project.

A Disease for the Affluent

The 1990s were a quieter decade for cinematic representations of cancer in India. However, filmmakers returned to the theme at the turn of the century, developing narrative concerns with disclosure in new ways. At the same time, these newer films, produced after economic liberalization, contrast with those of earlier decades in one important way: cancer seems to appear only in the lives of the wealthy. *Vaada Raha* (I promise), released in 2009, exemplifies this cinematic orientation. The film's hero, Dr. Dyanesh Chawla, goes by the transnationally legible name Duke. Duke exemplifies the fantasies of a world after India's economic liberalization; he moves across an opulent global space of clubs, designer clothes, and sports cars, transcending all regional boundaries. His wealth comes from his work as a brilliant cancer surgeon and researcher. After receiving a grant from the American Medical Association to continue his search for a cure, he proposes marriage to his girlfriend, Pooja, but before they can get married, he is paralyzed in a car accident. In a stark reversal of the conjugal sacrifices characterizing the films of earlier decades, Pooja abandons him over the phone, sending Duke spiraling into suicidal depression. Rehearsing the trope of the magical cancer patient, a child named Roshan (whose name translates as "light") brings sunshine into Duke's life: he draws open the curtains in Duke's hospital room and tells him cheery stories from the world outside. Like Anand and

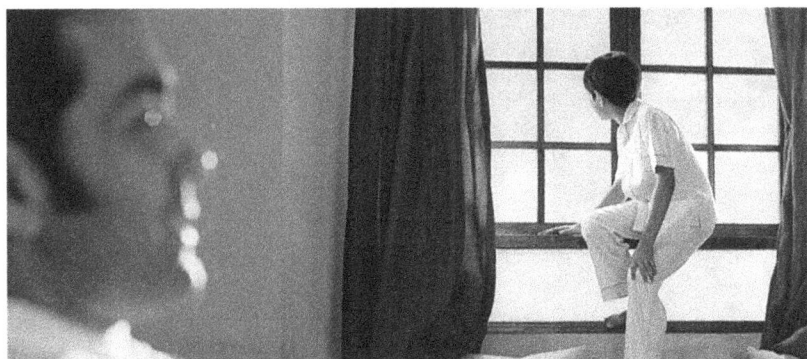

FIGURE 5.13 Still from *Vaada Raha* (2009). Roshan opens the windows, bringing light into Duke's life.

Milli, Roshan infects all around him with his hyperactive optimism. Sure enough, Duke's spirit is revived, and he returns to surgery and research, even discovering a cure for leukemia. However, his happiness is tempered when he learns that Roshan died moments before his discovery: he had been a leukemia patient all along and had hidden his diagnosis from Duke. The final scene of the film finds Duke reunited with Pooja and playing with his son, whom he has named after Roshan.

While *Vaada Raha* resembles *Anand* and *Milli* in resuscitating the trope of the magical cancer patient, its mise-en-scène of global opulence is a new development in the Indian cancer film. It is in keeping with broader trends at the turn of the century when Hindi cinema mutated into "Bollywood" and oriented itself toward national and transnational elites.[18] Critics and audiences alike punished *Vaada Raha* for having a narrative that seemed implausible, even within the generous allowances of fantasy afforded by the aesthetics of Hindi film. But the runaway success of *Waqt: The Race against Time* a few months later suggests that *Vaada Raha* might have fared better if it had cast more commercially reliable stars.

Waqt returned Amitabh Bachchan to the Hindi cancer film after his success in the genre in *Anand* and *Milli*. This time, however, Bachchan plays a cancer patient. *Waqt* is symptomatic of Bachchan's late career. After his work in *Anand* and *Milli*, Bachchan became synonymous with the heroic trope of the "angry young man" in Hindi films in the 1970s: he played violent, anti-authoritarian characters who channeled intense social discontentment. In contrast, in the years following India's liberalization, Bachchan has almost exclusively played the role of a wealthy patriarch—conformist and conser-

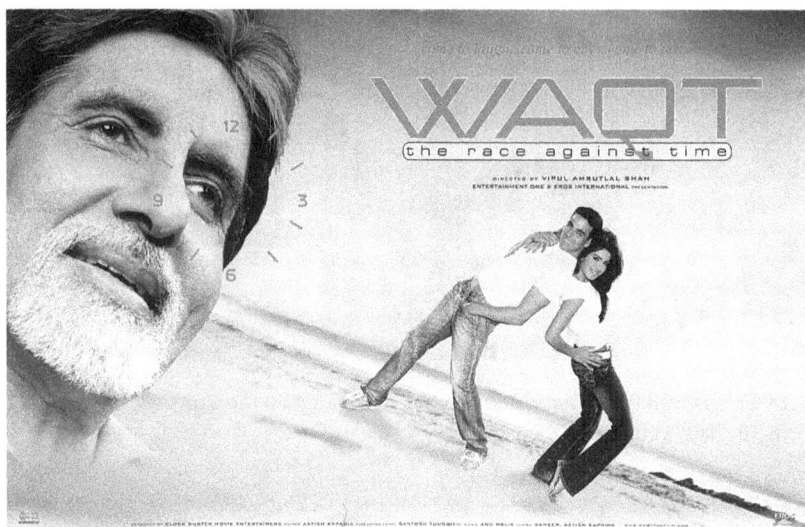

FIGURE 5.14 Film poster for *Waqt: The Race against Time* (2005). Image from Osianama Research Centre Archive, Library and Sanctuary, India.

vative in his social attitudes.[19] His role in *Waqt* is no exception. He plays Ishwarchand Thakur, a rich patriarch whose only vice is his excessive love for his profligate son, Aditya. After Aditya's marriage to his equally wealthy fiancée, Pooja, we find out that Ishwarchand has been hiding his terminal cancer diagnosis from Aditya; he did not want to dull the joy of his son's marriage. But as his disease progresses, Ishwarchand worries about Aditya's future. He banishes Aditya from his house to teach him to fend for himself. Remarkably, the banishment only extends to the house's physical walls, and Aditya continues to live in Ishwarchand's palatial outhouse. Yet, Ishwarchand is shattered by having to harden his heart against his son. To mend his fortunes, Aditya turns to a televised competitive game show and qualifies for the grand finale, nearing his goal to become a rich and successful actor. Ishwarchand is overjoyed and now has another reason to conceal his diagnosis: he does not want to distract Aditya from achieving success. But Aditya finds out about his father's diagnosis on the night of his performance. In his own act of self-sacrifice, he does not perform but begs the audience to pray for his father's health. The stakes of this sacrifice are low; the audience responds to his piety, and he wins the competition without having to perform. The family reunites moments before Ishwarchand's death, but he lives on as he can name his grandson after himself in his dying breath. The patriarch dies of cancer but, in his death, gifts his son his name and wealth.

With films like *Vaada Raha* and *Waqt*, we are far removed from the hints of progressive concerns in the films of the 1960s. In their single-minded focus on the reunification of wealthy families, they also move away from the films of the 1970s. That is, if social difference was the focus of the films in the 1960s, it remained implicit in the 1970s, even as it was pushed to the margins of narrative concern. Recall the opening scene of *Anand*, where Bachchan wandered around distraught in Bombay's slums, frustrated by his inability as a doctor to treat cancer among the poor. Also recall the closing scenes of *Ankhiyon Ke Jharakon Se*, where Lily's death led to Sachin's commitment to a philanthropic medical vocation in her memory. The 1970s films pushed social responsibility to the edges of narratives but did not completely dismiss the need for some social reform. After the turn of the century, however, the elision of class and collective suffering reached its apogee, and cancer as a disease seemed only to afflict the country's wealthy.

Indian cancer films have thus produced many visions of the normative. To summarize: In the 1960s, the first set of cancer films magnified disease onto the space of national sacrifice and reform. Through the 1970s, this outward magnification was inverted, as the genre drew inward to psychological dramas of cheerful resilience. In this second generation of cancer films, the object of sacrifice turned toward a proximal other—a lover or a friend—and their individualized distress. Finally, films about cancer after the turn of the century took flight from concerns about social inequity, narrativizing the importance of familial unity and stability as a response to cancer. Thus, over time, the cinematic imagination of cancer transformed from a concern with the nation and its citizens, to intimate psychological dramas, and finally to a world of affluent patriarchy.

Blurred Realties

If the star persona of Amitabh Bachchan—as it develops through *Anand*, *Milli*, and *Waqt*—is one way to synoptically arrange these shifting orientations of the Indian cancer film, the dynastic Dutt family is another. Sunil Dutt was one of Indian cinema's most well-known actors from the late 1950s to the 1980s. His breakthrough role was alongside Indian cinema's most highly regarded actress, Nargis, in the Oscar-nominated *Mother India*. Nargis and Sunil Dutt married soon after making the film, and their son— Sanjay Dutt—is now one of contemporary Indian cinema's most successful actors. Cancer intersects the biographical and cinematic lives of the Dutt family. In 1979, Nargis was diagnosed with pancreatic cancer and was flown

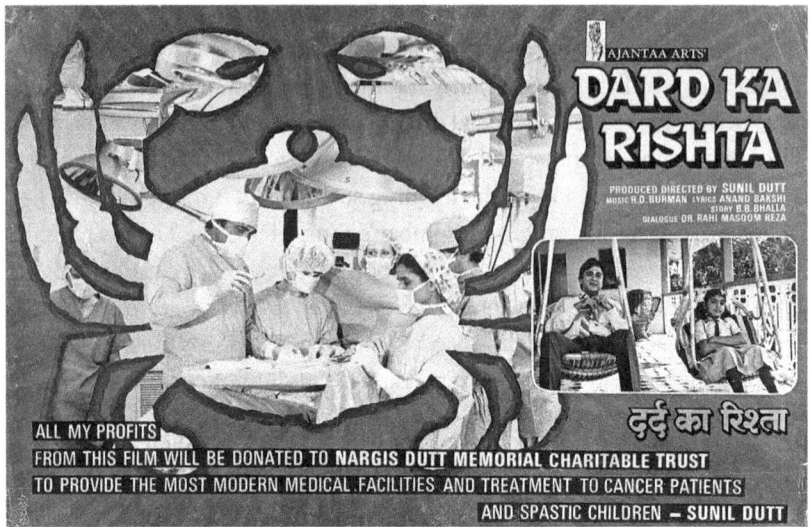

FIGURE 5.15 Film poster for *Dard Ka Rishta* (1982). Image from Osianama Research Centre Archive, Library and Sanctuary, India.

to Sloan Kettering Memorial Hospital in New York for treatment. After two years of treatment in New York, she returned to India, only for her condition to worsen. Sanjay Dutt flew her team of doctors from New York to India, but she passed away before they could treat her again.[20] Through the course of Nargis's treatment, Sunil Dutt made his first and last foray into film direction with *Dard Ka Rishta* (A relation of pain).

Released in 1982, the film narrativizes Dutt's distress at his wife's death the previous year. During Nargis's treatment, Dutt had resolved to start an Indian cancer foundation in her name: *Dard Ka Rishta* begins with a title card announcing the foundation and promising to it Dutt's earnings from the film. In the film Dutt plays Dr. Ravi, who is married to a cancer re-searcher, Anuradha. They live in New York and work at Sloan Kettering. The film begins with Dutt receiving a job offer from Tata Memorial, the fa-mous public cancer hospital in Bombay. He is resolved to go, but Anuradha refuses to return to India because she does not believe she will have research facilities in Bombay comparable to those in New York. Echoing the films of the 1960s, her commitment to research is motivated by the leukemia diagno-sis and death of her young brother. Ravi sees the conundrum, telling Anu-radha: "You cannot betray your brother; I cannot betray my country." This becomes the film's "relation of pain": if exegetically the film is motivated by

Dutt's pain in separation from Nargis, diegetically it is transformed into Ravi and Anuradha's divorce. They are both committed to cancer, but the gap between treatment and research is irreconcilable. Exegesis and diegesis collapse again in the appearance of Dr. Edward Beattie as a character in the film. The famous physician who headed Sloan Kettering from 1966 to 1983 had treated Nargis.

Ravi returns to India to help the Indian poor at Tata Memorial. The film text again blurs diegesis and exegesis. Over a series of montages of suffering among the Indian poor, Dutt proclaims that there can be no answer to cancer unless "our socialism leaves the grasp of our constitution and enters the sunlight of our country; that is the only cure." Dutt nonetheless struggles against all odds to save as many patients as he can. Here, the film introduces the character of a freedom fighter who had fought for India's decolonization. He comes to the hospital for Ravi's care and is diagnosed with treatable cancer. However, he refuses to go abroad for treatment until the poor in the country have the same opportunities for care; even though he has the means to receive treatment, he will die. He threatens the political establishment in a direct address to camera: "I will die, and my death will haunt the parliament houses of this country."

In watching *Dard Ka Rishta*, audiences would have known of the real-life subtexts of the film. The film is informed not only by Nargis's death but also by the controversial decision to send the Indian president Sanjiva Reddy to Edward Beattie at Sloan Kettering for treatment in 1977.[21] During a routine checkup, doctors at AIIMS discovered a small lesion in the president's lungs. A panel of twelve doctors at the institute referred the president's treatment to Dr. Beattie—the same physician who would later treat Nargis—rather than treating him in India. This decision not only was criticized by India's leading oncologists but also troubled the new prime minister, Morarji Desai. In somewhat of a panic, Desai sanctioned the quick import of two linear particle accelerators, the most expensive radiotherapy machine at that time, with each machine costing about 2 crore rupees (38 crores postinflation, or about US$5 million). An angry editorial in the *Economic and Political Weekly* announced that ten cobalt radiotherapy machines could have been imported for the same price.[22] Cobalt machines were arguably equally effective in treating cancer and would have been able to treat about three times as many patients as the linear accelerators in the same time. It was shortly after this controversy that the government announced the decision to set up a dedicated cancer hospital at AIIMS, the site of my fieldwork described in the first chapter. In a fascinating postscript to this story, Lawrence Cohen con-

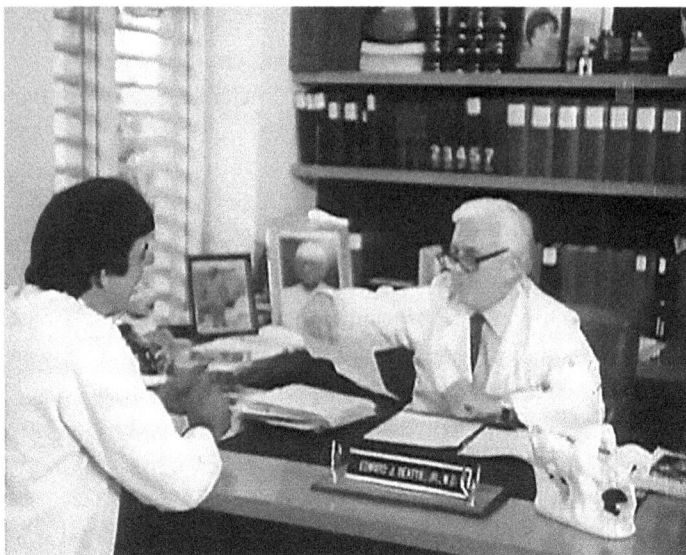

FIGURE 5.16 Still from *Dard Ka Rishta* (1982). Dr. Edward Beattie from Sloan Kettering Hospital in New York tells Ravi (Sunil Dutt) of a job offer for Ravi from Tata Memorial Hospital. Behind the desk stands a mounted picture of the Indian president Neelam Sanjiva Reddy, who had recently been treated by Dr. Beattie.

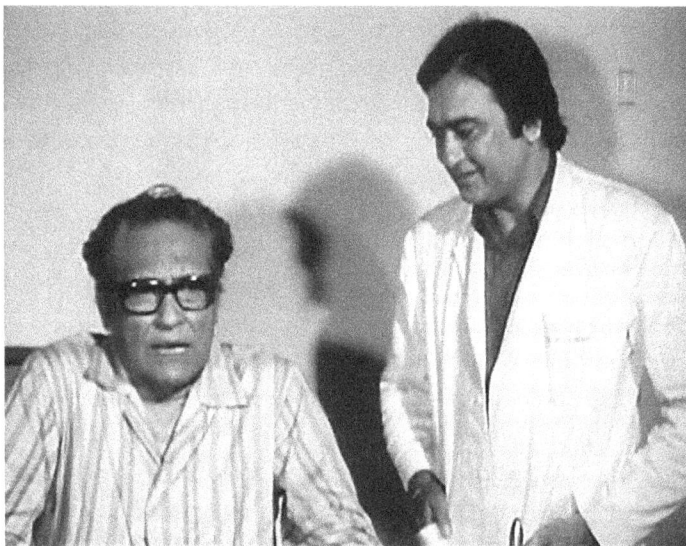

FIGURE 5.17 Still from *Dard Ka Rishta* (1982). A freedom fighter tells Ravi that he would rather die than receive cancer treatment that is unavailable to other citizens.

trasts the consternation around Reddy's foreign operation with the absence of controversy around Sonia Gandhi's visit abroad for cancer treatment.[23] In 2011, Gandhi, the leader of the Congress Party, traveled to the United States for a procedure to treat her cervical cancer. But this time, unlike with Sanjiva Reddy, Gandhi's visit caused little dismay in the media. Instead, reporting focused on the fact that her doctor was a nonresident Indian, celebrating his personal triumphant arc as he had transcended the disadvantage of his birth in a small Indian village.

Thus, while *Dard Ka Rishta* echoes the concerns about national sacrifice pervasive in cancer films before its own time, it also catalyzed a specific, contemporaneous alarm in the 1980s with the perceived failure of Indian hospitals to treat the disease. Two decades later, cancer and disease would return transformed to the forefront of the Dutt family's cinematic concerns. In the 2003 film *Munna Bhai M.B.B.S.*—one of the biggest box-office successes of the last two decades—Sanjay Dutt plays the role of a gangster-turned-doctor. Although Sunil Dutt had retired from cinema, he returned to play Sanjay's on-screen father, who wants his son to become a selfless doctor for the poor. Unwilling to disappoint his father, Munna pretends to be one and creates a fake charitable hospital in his father's name. However, Munna is found out and is ostracized by his father. Determined to make amends, Munna enrolls in a "real" medical college. He quickly rises to fame as a student because of his almost magical ability to cure patients with a hug, a method of comfort taught to him by his mother. The film becomes a tussle between the unfeeling profession of biomedicine personified by the college's dean, Dr. Asthana, and Munna's unconventional method of compassionate healing. The test of the two paradigms appears in the form of a depressed young cancer patient, Zaheer. Munna brings comfort to Zaheer, who comes to believe Munna is endowed with a magical gift. In his dying breath he looks to Munna for a cure, but Munna cannot bring him back to life. Instead, Zaheer dies while encircled by Munna's magical hug. Munna is devastated by this failure and leaves the college, much to Dr. Asthana's joy. But another patient in a vegetative state returns to life to vouch for Munna's goodness, convincing Dr. Asthana of his folly.

The bigenerational Dutt films—*Dard Ka Rishta* and *Munna Bhai M.B.B.S.* —capture two broad trajectories of Indian cancer films. On the one hand, *Dard Ka Rishta* is an example of melodramatic alignment of cancer as simultaneously a public and private ethical crisis. The disease demands sacrifices, and in Indian cinema of an early postcolonial period, the sacrifices to the new nation-state took precedence over the desires of immediate kin.

On the other, *Munna Bhai M.B.B.S.* exemplifies a cinematic turn inward to consider the disease's effect on individual interiorities. The ethical crisis produced by cancer shifts from concerns with nation and citizenship to a matter of interpersonal compassion. Thus, in its many, varied representations of cancer, Indian film reveals how different historical moments inflect aesthetic concerns. In each of these films, cancer plays the role of a transformative agent. But the object of transformation is an ever-shifting target: from the nation, to a proximate other, to the concerns of postliberalization wealth and the retrenchment of traditional family values in a time of social change.

The Felicity of Melodrama

I was drawn to exploring films about cancer when I found public health experts and physicians demeaning them for presenting a bleak picture of life with the disease. These elite experts and physicians believed that the overwhelming sense of melodramatic pathos in Hindi cinema was detrimental to the psychological well-being of their patients. My reading of these films takes exactly the opposite tack. Rather than castigate pathos and melodrama, I find them to be aesthetic choices felicitous to imagining and magnifying the stakes of ethical crises in social relations around cancer. For example, in the early decades after decolonization, the disease set the stage for protagonists to sacrifice themselves for the greater good of the nation. In the middle postcolonial period, films retreated from this preoccupation with public responsibility into familial psychodramas about hope and despair after diagnosis. And after economic liberalization, films further departed from their prior pedagogical impulses toward social good, and cancer appeared only in the celluloid lives of the elite and as reinforcing "traditional" values.

For each of these films, then, the aesthetic conventions of the melodrama opened several possibilities for imagining the pathos of the disease. Many films narrativized how kin cared for each other by taking on the burden of concealing the diagnosis. To do so, they took recourse to the mode of melodrama to narrativize how this concealed knowledge came to reside in the bodies of protagonists, eventually destroying them or driving them to the point of madness. Others told stories of how men fighting the disease sacrificed themselves while women silently bore the weight and consequences of these heroic sacrifices long after the men's death. Through the narrative device of cancer, these films took up melodrama's preoccupation with the long-standing suffering of virtuous female protagonists. Yet other films explored whether patients could transcend their suffering through a heightening of optimism and hope, deploying melodrama's ability to dramatize excesses of affect. Adopting the conventions of melodrama, they took on the ambitious task of magnifying the stakes of the disease—the failed promise of decolonization, the propriety of gender roles, the decline in family values, the duties of care placed upon kin, and so on. And in their resolutions, often achieved through the death of a protagonist, each film offered moral lessons about how to transcend the trouble cancer introduced into social life. The disease—and the crisis it produces in social relations—became a way to map personal subjectivities onto public imaginaries, connecting the two in surprising yet historically contingent ways. At the same time, this mapping was rarely complete or resolved. The eruptive presence of excess always threatened the surface of the text in filmic melodramas, a reminder to us of the dangers of abstracting the disease for the purposes of didactic, moral pedagogy.

The films about cancer I am most drawn to share one impulse with the cancer memoirs I find most compelling: they "capture something that is fundamental and generally unacknowledged—that the experience of illness and dying lies beyond our ability to describe it fully in language or to impart to it coherence or expressive form."[24] It is precisely these moments of uncertainty and hesitancy that are the felicity of certain aesthetic accounts of cancer, especially those in the early postcolonial representations of the disease. For example, films such as *Satyakam, Dil Ek Mandir*, and *Saathi* never fully resolve the ethical contradictions they set up in their narratives. In these early films, cancer offered male protagonists a chance to sacrifice themselves for the sake of the nation. And as the disease aligned with other kinds of social failures—the stigmatization of widows, bureaucratic graft, oppressive feudal customs, limited biomedical infrastructures—curing or transcending cancer similarly aligned neatly with a range of social reformist impulses.

However, this neat alignment could not obscure deeper, unresolved contradictions. As men sacrificed themselves, the costs of their sacrifice fell upon their wives. These sacrifices imposed a durative suffering on women, who were allowed brief moments of melodramatic eruption in which to verbalize this suffering. But mostly, women testified to this erasure through displays of emotive excess and embodied pathos. Caught within a structure of misrecognition in which they were fated to silence, they performed hysteria, self-harm, or self-erasure. Thus, if cancer afforded men opportunities of visibility and magnification, the structure of its filmic narratives disallowed this equal footing to women, whose sacrifice took the form of self-erasure.

The easy metaphoric alignments of cancer with social reform always turned out to incur disproportionately gendered costs. Finally, then, I read these films as aesthetic reflections on the vast chasms the disease opens between subjectivity and its fulfillment, between experience and expression.

By narrativizing these deep contradictions and crises without fully resolving them, these early postcolonial films revealed the dangers of deploying cancer to proselytize a univocal message. In these early films, readers and audiences are offered a glimpse, however brief, into the durability and irresolvability of doubts and suspicions that closely haunt the experience of life-threatening illness. And it is precisely this openness to irresolution and contradiction that is lost in films of the last two decades, in which cancer serves to discipline protagonists into proper family values and gender roles, proselytizing cheer and optimism in response to the disease.

6

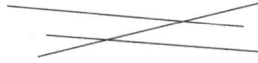

ENDURANCE

Endurance is not the work of overcoming adversity, of moving on or moving elsewhere, but the practices of making do in a protracted moment of dire and even
life-threatening uncertainty that seems so relentless it becomes ordinary.
—Zoë Wool, "In-Durable Sociality"

This book has been an exploration of my interlocutors' many experiments
with social relations through which they found ways to live with or alongside a cancer diagnosis. Cancer awakened doubts and skepticisms about social relations, articulating past vulnerabilities with present duress. To grapple with these doubts, my interlocutors staked models of pain, managed
speech about the disease, and experimented with ways to absorb past histories into the present. This is not to say that these experiments were always
successful: they took shape under conditions of social and economic constraint that continuously threatened to exhaust capacities for enduring the
disease. In what follows, I describe the ethical force of this will to endure,
in circumstances where pathways to collectivization and health care rights
were not readily at hand.

In recent years, anthropologists have been troubled by a perceived disciplinary obsession with suffering.[1] For example, Joel Robbins regrets that in
the last three decades, suffering has become anthropology's central preoccu-

pation and guiding rationale.[2] He is critical of this turn because he believes it frames suffering as *the* fundamental substrate of all human experience, erasing the proper subject of anthropological inquiry—cultural difference. To redress this disciplinary mistake, Robbins asks for a redirection of anthropological attention away from suffering and violence and toward social projects of hope, empathy, and care. I raise Robbins's criticisms here because this book might well be accused of perpetuating an anthropological fascination with the suffering of others. In its pages, projects of radical social transformation are hard to discern. Indeed, when I write of hope, optimism, empathy, and care, I do so to point to their limits and false promises. Instead, my interest here is with the durable consequences of long-standing precarity and the slow, chronic violence of cancer that leaves few opportunities for survival, recovery, or transformation. Do I then present a picture of my interlocutors' life as void of the possibility of ethical action, a problem that Robbins finds characteristic of contemporary anthropology? In describing practices oriented to endurance in the present, rather than transformation in the future, do I portray my interlocutors as passive bystanders to their fate? Indeed, as anthropologists partial to Robbins's critique have asked, "What is the point in yet another description of the capacity of humans to feel pain and suffer?"[3] This is a problem well worth discussion because its concerns extend beyond disciplinary anthropology, implicating allied fields (journalism, photography, and humanitarian work) whose practices similarly aim to respond to social marginalization.[4]

In responding to this critique, I share its concern about anthropology's possibly voyeuristic attraction to suffering, but I do not agree with the clear lines such a critique draws between suffering and flourishing.[5] Recent critiques, including but not limited to those of Robbins, distinguish between an anthropology attentive to suffering, and one that is attuned to well-being, ethical flourishing, and the so-called good life. Such a division misses something I have had occasion to describe many times in my ethnography: the close interlocking of care and violence, of empathy and neglect, and of hope and exhaustion, all of whose paths ran through each other in everyday practices of tending to cancer. More specifically, valorizing hope and optimism misses the pervasive cruelty of urging resilience as a response to cancer, in circumstances where recovery and survival are an ever-receding horizon. I argue, then, that separating descriptions of suffering and violence from those of hope and empathy sets up a false divide between trajectories of human experience that are often inextricably tied. Trying to distinguish the two zones of human experience misses how optimism and hope do not always ease suffering but are often the very conditions of their possibility.[6] For example, in tracking palliative cancer care research, I found a recurrent call to operationalize Indian capacities for resilience in order to withstand pain caused by infrastructural neglect. In tracking how cancer entered conjugal relationships, I found practices of care tied to forms of violence in ways that blurred the lines between the two. In tracking the generic tendencies of cancer memoirs, I described their injunction to greet cancer with joy, as an opportunity to find a better life and expiate past sins. These injunctions were suffused with the cruel promise that if patients learned to love their disease, they would easily transcend suffering. And in exploring films about cancer, I found that their resolutions transformed suffering into neat moral lessons about how to find happiness and optimism in the face of death, looking away from their socioeconomic conditions of possibility. In these and many other ways, I was struck by how projects of hope, empathy, and care were often the very preconditions for the presence and continuance of suffering, rather than its redress. Often, promises of a way out—of recovering a "good life" or achieving a "good death"—were premised on fantasies that had little to do with the durability of distress in the everyday lives of my interlocutors.

It is difficult for me, then, to reconcile my ethnography with the anthropological demand to explore projects of hope, separating out such projects from those that are steeped in violence and suffering. Rather, my aim in this book has been to explore how my interlocutors made the present livable, rejecting calls to transcend the disease through the sheer force of optimism and personal will. Without recourse to collective projects that offered radical social transformation and health care rights, without often even the possibility of surviving and recovering from the disease, my interlocutors carved out strategies through which they negotiated care, kin, and bodily damage in the present. I suggest that for anthropology to find its ethical ground, turning away from these modes of endurance would miss an entire terrain of action and inventiveness that has been the focus of this book—projects that do not presuppose hope but that nevertheless strive to imagine a livable life. Such projects ask us to pause a moment in our construction of what ethical action in the face of constrained possibilities might look like. While anthropologists oriented toward hope look for ethical projects seeking to transform the present in search of a better life, my effort here has been to think of ethics not as such a project of becoming different but, rather, as a durative confrontation with circumstances and constraints as they are. Such a picture of ethics reveals the intense effort often required to stay the same, in conditions of slow and steady deterioration. In so doing, they call our attention to what Sandra Laugier calls an ethics of ordinary realism—an ethics attentive to what is right before our eyes—everyday projects of the maintenance of fragile worlds on the verge of collapse.[7]

I find it important to pay attention to such ethical projects of endurance not only because they reject false promises of hope but also because they are acutely diagnostic of the force and form of the violence they confront. In their response, projects of endurance reveal a particular slow violence, one directed at slowly exhausting capacities for life, rather than dramatically taking life.[8] In his Collège de France lectures, Michel Foucault describes the historical relation of life and politics as a movement from an experience of the epidemic to the endemic. If in the Middle Ages, state power focused on the management of mass deaths because of fast-spreading and ever-looming epidemics, from the eighteenth century, it came to be concerned with another kind of threat—illnesses that were endemic. Endemics, in Foucault's description, are not spectacles of epidemic catastrophe and mass-produced deaths, but rather a permanent threat to life that saps at a population's strength. Avoiding the framing of cancer as something particularly new and distinct from diseases that have come before, I have developed the idea of cancer as endemic rather than epidemic. Throughout this book, I have suggested that cancer—a disease synonymous with crisis and rupture—is also a matter of slow, chronic, and endemic concern. Rather than distinguish between a catastrophic illness event and an endemic one, I take my cue from my ethnography to think of the two together—of crises that might become endemic, of catastrophes that challenge without entirely eluding everyday strategies of endurance.[9]

In her analysis of the persistence of colonial violence in the present, Ann Stoler offers an analytic of power in terms of duress.[10] Thinking of power as duress draws attention to its elusive presence in everyday life and intimate socialities. Thinking of duress helps suspend an already clear sense of knowing what the relation between power and vulnerability looks like. In my work, thinking of the constrained life chances of my informants as duress helps to explain how a long history of marginalization and failed state policies attenuated capacities of endurance. Throughout my ethnography, there were few moments in which state failures revealed themselves in dramatic gestures. There were few moments in which I could easily identify, for example, how an act of denying care resulted directly in cancer or death. Rather, violence unfolded in the shape of slow-moving queues, as treatments delayed rather than denied, as intimate hostilities masquerading as care, and as circumscribed possibilities of speech demanding strategic concealments. In these and many other ways, forms of violence, inextricably tied to care and empathy, were hardly predictable in advance; they appeared only in their sedimented effects on bodies in pain and the burning out of the will to persevere. In response, endurance unfolded here as an attunement, attachment, and attention to the present: as strategies of speech, as carefully choreographed acts of giving and seeking care, as the work of remaining within fraught kinship ties, and as aesthetic confrontations with the fragmentations of grief.[11] The promise of such an ethics of endurance was not one of recovery or transcendence, but rather of a survival and persistence in the present, predicated on grasping how critical illness reverberated through precarious socialities.

The testimony of R. Anuradha, a cancer patient who sought treatment at AIIMS during the time of my fieldwork there, offers a paracommentary on my own description of the ethics of endurance. Anuradha has published two books, one prose and one poetry, that recount her life with cancer. Her description bears re-presentation here, even as it is mediated through my translation from Hindi to English and distorted through my excerpting of passages.

The idioms of the body are strange
Its language is strange, . . .
When it most needs to speak
It becomes silent
Amid many people
Gathered around to talk
In that gathering, about the body
I became silent
Its volubility wants solitude, silence . . .
Because for the body to speak
Is to lose language[12]

Relations break in a few words . . .
The cup of life
Slips from our hands
Breaks
Shatters into fragments
Becomes wounds
That are later filled
Doctors in hospitals change
Their referrals change
Prescriptions change

Dosages change
Sometimes we
change doctors
But don't you change,
pain
Be by my side.[13]

R. Anuradha's writings capture with stunning precision a curious juxtaposition expressed by many people I spoke to—a juxtaposition of the constancy of pain with the inconstancy of social relations. People, doctors, referrals, and dosages change, while crowds, kin, and neighbors gather and disperse. The world, fragile as glass, fragments. Her description of striving to live in such circumstances offers a glimpse into the deep doubt about social relations in the shadow of cancer and its accompanying pain. But at the same time, there is an unwavering realization in her work that however inadequate, it is through social relations that one might find pain's amelioration:

To stay silent is wrong
To sit silent is also wrong
Don't become silent
Don't be silent
Speak
That we are not just those
Who have been cut by surgery
Burnt by radiation
Poisoned by medicine
Plagued
By loneliness, emptiness
Even when pain brings us to tears
We must be obstinate.[14]

Thus, even as pain jeopardizes social relations, even as it demands silence, it is also obstinately voluble. It is to this double command—to respect the intractability of pain at the same time as tending to it—that palliative care physicians strove to respond. Cancer pain came into being in Delhi through the process of doctors and patients struggling, often unsuccessfully, to formulate an agreement on its etiologies. To ameliorate it, physicians offered both proximal and distal models for its apprehension. While in practice they were expert at diagnosing and treating the condition through touch and sight, in research, their speculations offered more distal pathways—routed through

India's colonial past and postcolonial present. Each model offered a different vision of empathy—a distinct way of relating to the ubiquity and intransigency of cancer pain. The psychosocial model of pain I found in my fieldwork was an expert hypothesis about the social worlds in which cancer appeared, and how such worlds might contribute to or ease suffering.

Pain, then, is a paradigmatic scene of the practices of endurance that concern me here. Living with it, alongside it, or intervening into it evidences an attunement and attachment to the present, to work and live within social relations at their most brittle and fragile. This is not to say that there was something beautiful or worthwhile in enduring pain for pain's sake. I do not want to resurrect theories that suffering might be a proper ground for the body's moral potentiality, as some theological traditions have it.[15] Rather, describing pain as a scene of endurance highlights the effort to live within social relations at their most delicate moments, alongside the constant possibility of the denial of recognition, care, and empathy. Enduring pain involved seeking recognition that was sometimes offered, as often as it was withheld. For example, for cancer care NGO workers, responding to pain meant understanding the kinship worlds and neighborhood dynamics of the patients and families under their care. Within families, the seeking and giving of care after a cancer diagnosis often involved grappling with past histories of domestic violence. Locating ethics in efforts to withstand and respond to pain is especially crucial in such contexts where pain persists, despite injunctions to transcend it and despite the best efforts of the physicians I worked with to declare their hospital a "pain-free" zone.

The striving to endure pain, then, involved asking for recognition, risking misrecognition. Pain's ebbs and flows were often revelatory of the limits and possibilities of recovery and care offered by already fragile social worlds. Let me turn again to Anuradha's poetry:

I contain
great depths,
And great emptiness,
Loose,
Like hair,
Brittle are my ribs,
Fill them,
With the touch of your sight,
Like heated irons,
Always in freezing storms of pain,

With the fever of your soft hands,
Cool me down.[16]

Relations are not bricks
that mortar can make solid
put in a mold, dried and fired
stamped with the mark of the maker
to become a wall.[17]

Anuradha captures here one of my central arguments: that confrontations with cancer's pain were always confrontations with the fragility of social relations around cancer. At the beginning of this book, I described how a construction worker rebuilt his home to ease his wife's cancer pain. He had borrowed materials to carve out ornate moldings, framed photographs of their past, and repainted the walls, hoping through these gestures to construct the possibility of a shared future. But relations were not always so dependable. Efforts to endure required a constant negotiation of social relations, testing them for points of strength and vulnerability, determining when they could be depended on and when they might break under the weight of the diagnosis.

If the experience of pain was a paradigmatic scene of endurance, concealment was its mode of practical experimentation. In their many forms, concealments were never a stable or uniform set of practices, but constantly shifted in relation to different people and at different moments in the illness trajectory. But in each instance, strategic concealments (as well as tentative disclosures) revealed how in the wake of a cancer diagnosis, patients, families, and physicians trafficked in the possibilities of "as-ifs," multiplying the ways in which the disease was expressed in social practices. Sometimes, concealment was a form of care, performing hope in the face of imminent death. At other times, it was a way to safeguard oneself from dangerous relations. In each of these ways, concealment opened a space of the subjunctive, a brief respite from the real, even when such respite never really escaped the grasp of the actual. To think of concealment as experiments in endurance is to recognize the unpredictable ways agency might appear in times of duress and social fragility. By concealing their diagnosis from some, disclosing strategically to others, my interlocutors worked to maintain social relations, safeguarding a present on the verge of coming undone. Concealment, then, was an act directed at surviving in the present, not at flourishing in the future. As Clara Han puts it in the context of her work in Chile, concealing often reveals the moral energy required for endurance.[18]

Further, to pay attention to an ethics directed at endurance is also to understand the harms that people might do to each other, in precisely the same gestures they invent to survive. In consonance with my work here, Zoë Wool coins the expression "in-durance" to point to a mode of life lived in precisely such a relentless present, whose futures are uncertain and hardly secure.[19] Thinking of concealment and strategic disclosures as practices of endurance offers a troubling insight: that efforts to endure sometimes foreclose efforts directed toward social transformation. Indeed, in its negative sense, certain practices of endurance interrupt the formation of "biosocial" collectives that have become of interest to medical anthropologists in recent years. To elaborate, Adriana Petryna and Nikolas Rose and Carlos Novas developed the concept of "biological citizenship" to capture a new relation between disease and the claiming of rights that share biological conditions.[20] And as Deborah Heath, Rayna Rapp, and Karen-Sue Taussig's nuanced formulation of "genetic citizenship" captures, these redefinitions of the social often lead to unanticipated alliances, redefining participatory citizenship in the process.[21] In part, Cansupport has sought to join these global forms of biosociality, incorporating many of the forms of cancer collectives elsewhere in the world, adopting global vocabularies of "Walk for Life" and "Survivor Days." But at the same time as Cansupport made a claim upon the public sphere, the everyday work of the NGO pointed to the difficulties of producing such collectivities, and concealment proved an obdurate obstacle to collectivization in an activist sense. I do not, then, want to claim a sense of political virtue for projects of endurance. Tending to maintain the present, such practices were often difficult grounds on which to build projects of radical social change. At the same time, I think it bears repeating that the play of disclosures and concealments I described were intensely social and relational, demanding a diagnosis and confrontation with the present. Even if their models of sociality do not fit preexisting templates of "biosocial" collectivity or offer a transparent vision of the "good," they are no less worthy of anthropological attention and understanding. Such practices urge us to assess the limits of our scholarly vocabularies, and of the purchase of an analytics of biosociality across different and uneven social terrains.

If pain was a paradigmatic scene of endurance and concealment exemplary of its enactment, the aesthetic accounts I examined transformed endurance into virtue. That is, in contrast to my ethnographic work, where endurance was an ever-unfinished and often unrewarding struggle, many films and memoirs about cancer sought and found resolutions that filled endurance with positive meaning. By being resilient, they claimed, the social could again be made whole. By the sheer dint of personal will, optimism, or sacrifice, the failing postcolonial nation could be reformed, traditional family values could be restituted, or past moral failures atoned. Memoirs promised restitution if patients learned to live more authentic lives, relinquishing their pessimism. Films resolved social crises through the death of the patient, offering in that gesture an ethical pedagogy of how to transcend suffering. As such, the generic conventions of aesthetic narratives offered a way out of the "in-durability" of endurance. Exploring these ways out offers an analytic counterpoint to the strategies of endurance that run through the rest of the book. These resolved aesthetic accounts put into sharp relief the irresolution of the everyday, and the ethical force and demand of endurance when such pathways to transcendence are not easily at hand.

In sum, by thinking through pain, concealment, and aesthetic resolutions, a guiding aim of this book has been to track the many strategies of endurance that my interlocutors experimented with so that they could live with or alongside the disease. Zoë Wool and Julie Livingston give the name "afterworlds" to places where life comes unhinged from the pervasive hope of a better future.[22] Pushed to their brink by long-standing political and economic violence, afterworlds are often defined by the inescapable threat of the exhaustion of life. In such conditions, Wool and Livingston argue that projects directed at survival are often as difficult as projects to transcend the present and become otherwise. In consonance, my description of an ethics of endurance in this book has evidenced the effort of my interlocutors to remain attached to the present in conditions hostile to their survival, without recourse to fantasies of what might have been, or what might come to be.

While such a description of endurance might present its dynamics as an unmoving stillness, my hope is that it appears as a practice of responsive plasticity, where strategies of life are continuously invented to resist the duress of exhaustion. In their recent work, João Biehl and Peter Locke approach the global aftermath of the breakdown of social movements by looking for new projects directed at ethical fulfillment, however indiscernible and muted they might be.[23] They urge anthropologists to witness such efforts to live with, subvert, and elude knowledge and power, and to express world-altering desires even when such desires are impossible to fulfill. Doing so, they suggest, expands our conceptualization of ethical "becoming," revealing "the plastic power of people and the intricate problematics of how to live alongside, through, and despite the profoundly constraining effects of social, structural, and material forces, which are themselves plastic."[24] My impulse here departs from theirs to look for new social collectives, but it joins their effort to show that projects that strive to adapt to ever-shifting dynamics of constraint must in their response also be unfinished and plastic. That is, I have hoped here to describe the plasticity of endurance, its always unfinished work, and the inventiveness required to survive, persist, and retain form under impress of slow and chronic duress. Such an understanding of endurance—as a struggle to remain in the present—takes as its ethical material not an effort to transform the world but the careful and challenging work of maintaining a world under chronic threat. I turn again, and for the final time, to R. Anuradha to capture this effort of endurance to hold on to life as it is, especially in circumstances in which it is inclined to slip away:

This sand
is slipping fast
This fist
clench it hard
Grasped
a little will remain
wet
in sweaty hands
Open
fists hold no sand.[25]

NOTES

INTRODUCTION

1 Susan Sontag, *Illness as Metaphor* (New York: Farrar, Straus and Giroux, 1978).

2 Adam Seligman, Robert Weller, Michael Puett, and Bennett Simon, *Ritual and Its Consequences: An Essay on the Limits of Sincerity* (Oxford: Oxford University Press, 2008), 19; Vaibhav Saria, "To Be Some Other Name: The Naming Games That Hijras Play," *South Asia Multidisciplinary Academic Journal*, no. 12 (2015): 1–16.

3 Veena Das, "The Dreamed Guru: The Entangled Lives of the Amil and the Anthropologist," in *The Guru in South Asia*, ed. Jacob Copeman and Aya Ikegame (Abingdon, UK: Routledge, 2012), 144–66.

4 Byron J. Good et al., "In the Subjunctive Mode: Epilepsy Narratives in Turkey," *Social Science and Medicine* 38, no. 6 (1994): 835–42; Jerome S. Bruner, *Actual Minds, Possible Worlds* (Cambridge, MA: Harvard University Press, 1986), 26; Veena Das, *Affliction: Health, Disease, Poverty* (New York: Fordham University Press, 2015), 141.

5 Seligman, Weller, Puett, and Simon, *Ritual and Its Consequences.*

6 Cecilia Van Hollen, "Handle with Care: Rethinking the Rights versus Culture Dichotomy in Cancer Disclosure in India," *Medical Anthropology Quarterly* 32, no. 1 (2018): 59–84.

7 Mary-Jo DelVecchio Good, Byron J. Good, Cynthia Schaffer, and Stuart E. Lind, "American Oncology and the Discourse on Hope," *Culture, Medicine and Psychiatry* 14, no. 1 (1990): 59–79; Van Hollen, "Handle with Care."

8 Rayna Rapp, "The Thick Social Matrix for Bioethics: Anthropological Approaches," in *Bioethics in Cultural Contexts*, ed. Marcus Well, Dietmar Mieth, and Christoph Rehmann-Sutter (Dordrecht: Springer Netherlands, 2006), 341–51.

9 Sarah Pinto, *Where There Is No Midwife: Birth and Loss in Rural India* (New York: Berghahn Books, 2008), 189–208.

10 Anne-Lise François, *Open Secrets: The Literature of Uncounted Experience* (Stanford, CA: Stanford University Press, 2008).

11 In this sense, acts such as concealment are ethical in the sense that they are not a rupture of the habitual, a flight from the many conscious and unselfconscious acts that make up the terrain of everyday life. Rather, acts of concealment "re-

mind us that in the face of the precariousness of life the mundane rituals we evolve, the way we conceal knowledge that might hurt, the way we continue to secure routine, is what allows our lives with others to be regarded as ethical or unethical." Veena Das, "Ordinary Ethics," in *A Companion to Moral Anthropology*, ed. Didier Fassin (Malden, MA: Wiley-Blackwell, 2012), 133–49.

12 Elaine Scarry, *The Body in Pain: The Making and Unmaking of the World* (New York: Oxford University Press, 1985).

13 She lays bare the violence of the cognitive dissonance such discourses generate: celebrating survival but denigrating those who die; celebrating the self-agency to will oneself to being better but ignoring the constraints on agency that make it impossible to challenge the pervasive toxicity that produces cancer in the first place. Lochlann Jain, *Malignant: How Cancer Becomes Us* (Berkeley: University of California Press, 2013).

14 Juliet McMullin, "Cancer," *Annual Review of Anthropology* 45, no. 1 (2016): 253.

15 As one instance, Julie Livingston describes how pain runs through the experience of cancer in Botswana. Even as it is often unvocalized and hidden, it is crucial in bringing patients to the cancer ward, where it creates demands for care and responsiveness. Julie Livingston, *Improvising Medicine: An African Oncology Ward in an Emerging Cancer Epidemic* (Durham, NC: Duke University Press, 2012), 142–43.

16 Here I draw from Andrew McDowell's suggestion that a "symptom provides analytical ground to link the body to social, economic, and historical factors." Andrew McDowell, "Mohit's Pharmakon: Symptom, Rotational Bodies, and Pharmaceuticals in Rural Rajasthan," *Medical Anthropology Quarterly* 31, no. 3 (2017): 332–48. For other examples of how symptoms help reveal local worlds of diseases and their sociality, see João Biehl and Amy Moran-Thomas, "Symptom: Subjectivities, Social Ills, Technologies," *Annual Review of Anthropology* 38, no. 1 (2009): 267–88; Mary-Jo DelVecchio Good, Sandra Theresa Hyde, Sarah Pinto, and Byron J. Good, *Postcolonial Disorders* (Berkeley: University of California Press, 2008); Jocelyn Lim Chua, "The Register of 'Complaint': Psychiatric Diagnosis and the Discourse of Grievance in the South Indian Mental Health Encounter," *Medical Anthropology Quarterly* 26, no. 2 (2012): 221–40; Clara Han, "Symptoms of Another Life: Time, Possibility, and Domestic Relations in Chile's Credit Economy," *Cultural Anthropology* 26, no. 1 (2011): 7–32.

17 Amy Moran-Thomas, "Struggles for Maintenance: Patient Activism and Dialysis Dilemmas amidst a Global Diabetes Epidemic," *Global Public Health* 14, nos. 6–7 (2019): 1044–57.

18 See, for example, Leonidas C. Goudas et al., "The Epidemiology of Cancer Pain," *Cancer Investigation* 23, no. 2 (2005): 182–90.

19 That is, taking the global south as generative of theory and explanations clarifies questions elsewhere in the world. Jean Comaroff and John L. Comaroff, *Theory from the South: Or, How Euro-America Is Evolving toward Africa* (London: Paradigm, 2012).

20 For excellent discussions of this phenomenon, see Barbara Ehrenreich, "Wel-

come to Cancerland," *Harper's*, November 2001; Léa Pool and Ravida Din, *Pink Ribbons, Inc.* (First Run Features, 2012).

21 Harmala Gupta, "Easing the Burden," *Times of India*, October 17, 2011.

22 Gupta, "Easing the Burden."

23 Cherian Koshy, "The Palliative Care Movement in India: Another Freedom Struggle or a Silent Revolution?," *Indian Journal of Palliative Care* 15, no. 1 (2009): 20–23.

24 Felicia Marie Knaul et al., "Alleviating the Access Abyss in Palliative Care and Pain Relief—an Imperative of Universal Health Coverage: The Lancet Commission Report," *Lancet* 391, no. 10128 (2018): 1391–454.

25 American Cancer Society, "Access to Essential Pain Medicines Brief (2013 Data)" (Atlanta: American Cancer Society, 2016).

26 Um-e-Kulsoom Shariff, "An Epidemic of Pain in India," *New Yorker*, December 5, 2018; Justin Rowlatt, "Why Are So Many People Denied the Painkillers They Need?," BBC, May 21, 2018.

27 Keith Wailoo, *Pain: A Political History* (Baltimore: Johns Hopkins University Press, 2015); Jean E. Jackson, *"Camp Pain": Talking with Chronic Pain Patients* (Philadelphia: University of Pennsylvania Press, 2000).

28 For its first century, colonial rule tolerated tradition and even expressed some admiration for ritual demonstrations of bodily fortitude. From the mid-nineteenth century, however, later colonial rulers tended to find these rituals decadent and without scriptural authority, and thus open to colonial projects of reform. Lata Mani, "Production of an Official Discourse on 'Sati' in Early Nineteenth Century Bengal," *Economic and Political Weekly* 21, no. 17 (1986): 32–40.

29 In this, my understanding of humanitarianism comes closest to Saiba Varma's suggestion that "organizations that focus on psychosocial suffering do not hold out the promise of life as much as they provide limited techniques for living with suffering. Far from universally embraced, this latter gift raises questions about the worthiness of humanitarian endeavors in places of long-term suffering." Saiba Varma, "The Medical Net: Patients, Psychiatrists and Paper Trails in the Kashmir Valley" (PhD diss., Cornell University, 2013).

30 David Holmes, "A Disease of Growth," *Nature* 521, no. 7551 (2015): S2–S3; T. Luzzati, A. Parenti, and T. Rughi, "Economic Growth and Cancer Incidence," *Ecological Economics* 146 (2018): 381–96.

31 Judith Fletcher-Brown, "India's Putting Economic Growth above All Else—and Thousands of Women Are Dying as a Result," *Quartz India*, October 18, 2017; Charu Bahri, "How Cancer Has India in Its Grip," *Scroll.in*, June 11, 2015.

32 Lindsey A. Torre, Rebecca L. Siegel, Elizabeth M. Ward, and Ahmedin Jemal , "Global Cancer Incidence and Mortality Rates and Trends: An Update," *Cancer Epidemiology, Biomarkers and Prevention* 25, no. 1 (2016): 16–27; World Health Organization, "Global Cancer Rates Could Increase by 50% to 15 Million by 2020," 2013, https://www.who.int/mediacentre/news/releases/2003/pr27/en/.

33 American Cancer Society, "Cancer Facts and Figures" (Atlanta: American Cancer Society, 2011), 45.

34 P. Farmer et al., "Expansion of Cancer Care and Control in Countries of Low and Middle Income: A Call to Action," *Lancet* 376, no. 9747 (2010): 1186–93.

35 Amy-Moran Thomas investigates this mistake in her work in health care in Belize, asking a powerful question: Why did international public health efforts focus their energies on infectious diseases, when diabetes was the number one cause of death in the country? She goes on to reject the division between "communicable" and "non-communicable" diseases, presenting a category of "para-communicable" diseases, such as diabetes, demonstrating how diabetes *is* transmittable, not only from mother to child in the womb but also molecularly triggered by trauma, intergenerational histories of hunger, environmental toxins, pharmaceutical side effects, and other comorbidities that remain difficult to gauge. Amy Moran-Thomas, "Metabola: Chronic Disease and Damaged Life in Belize" (PhD diss., Princeton University, 2012).

36 For example, around the fear of antibiotic resistance in the 1940s and 1950s and around multi-drug-resistant tuberculosis in the 1990s. David Jones and Jeremy Greene, "The Decline and Rise of Coronary Heart Disease: Understanding Public Health Catastrophism," *American Journal of Public Health* 103, no. 7 (2013): 1207–18.

37 Carlo Caduff, *The Pandemic Perhaps: Dramatic Events in a Public Culture of Danger* (Berkeley: University of California Press, 2015), 32.

38 Ian Magrath, "Cancer in Low and Middle Income Countries," in *Health G20*, ed. Manuel Carballo (Sutton, UK: Pro-Brook, 2010).

39 Torre, Siegel, Ward, and Jemal, "Global Cancer Incidence and Mortality Rates and Trends."

40 International Agency for Research on Cancer, "Globocan 2018: All Cancers Fact Sheet," accessed December 7, 2019, http://gco.iarc.fr/today/data/factsheets/cancers/39-All-cancers-fact-sheet.pdf.

41 Livingston, *Improvising Medicine*, 33.

42 I refer here to the International Agency for Research on Cancer estimate that 1,157,294 new cancer cases in India accounted for 15 percent of 18,078,957 new cancer cases globally in 2018. J. Ferlay et al., *Global Cancer Observatory: Cancer Today* (Lyon, France: International Agency for Research on Cancer, 2018), accessed December 7, 2019, https://gco.iarc.fr/today.

43 Ferlay et al., *Global Cancer Observatory*, and "Trends over Time for All Sites and on Selected Sites of Cancer and Projection of Burden of Cancer," in *Three-Year Report of Population Based Cancer Registries 2012–2014*, ed. National Centre for Disease Informatics and Research, National Cancer Registry Programme, and Indian Council of Medical Research (Bangalore: ICMR, 2016), 125.

44 Mohandas K. Mallath et al., "The Growing Burden of Cancer in India: Epidemiology and Social Context," *Lancet Oncology* 15, no. 6 (2014): e205–e212.

45 Preet K. Dhillon et al., "The Burden of Cancers and Their Variations across the States of India: The Global Burden of Disease Study 1990–2016," *Lancet Oncology* 19, no. 10 (2018): 1289–306; R. A. Badwe, R. Dikshit, M. Laversanne, and F. Bray, "Cancer Incidence Trends in India," *Japanese Journal of Clinical Oncology* 44, no. 5 (2014): 401–7.

46　See Lucas Mueller's persuasive claim that global health researchers have for long been concerned with the problem of cancer in the developing world and that "global health advocates' recent calls to attend to an emergent cancer epidemic in these regions were only the latest effort in this long history." What has really changed, then, is not that there is a "new" interest in cancer, but rather specific configurations of knowledge that shape the type of interventions that unfold. Lucas M. Mueller, "Cancer in the Tropics: Geographical Pathology and the Formation of Cancer Epidemiology," *BioSocieties* 14, no. 4 (2019): 512–28.

47　Kavita Sivaramakrishnan lays out how the problem of top-down histories of health in the twentieth century (that focuses on how global organizations determined an infectious disease agenda) miss how local actors did not necessarily distinguish between "infectious" and "malignant" disease in such clear-cut terms, thus giving the lie to the narrative of the developmentalist chronology of infectious diseases followed by chronic disease. Kavita Sivaramakrishnan, "Global Histories of Health, Disease, and Medicine from a 'Zig-Zag' Perspective," *Bulletin of the History of Medicine* 89, no. 4 (2015): 700–704.

48　"Recurrence of Malignant Growths after Removal," *British Medical Journal* 1, no. 1423 (1888): 766; "Cancer among Vegetarians," *British Medical Journal* 2, no. 1436 (1888): 29.

49　"The Cancer Danger," *Times of India*, August 10, 1904.

50　"The Cancer Problem," *Times of India*, May 3, 1911.

51　"Malignant Disease in India," *British Medical Journal* 1, no. 3926 (1936): 718–19.

52　Vishwa Nath and Khem Singh Grewal, "Cancer in India," *Indian Journal of Medical Research* 23, no. 1 (1935): 149–90.

53　Frederick I. Hoffman, "Cancer in India, Persia and Ceylon," *Sankhyā: The Indian Journal of Statistics (1933–1960)* 2, no. 3 (1936): 281–306.

54　Kavita Sivaramakrishnan, *As the World Ages: Rethinking a Demographic Crisis* (Cambridge, MA: Harvard University Press, 2018), 79–83.

55　Sivaramakrishnan, *As the World Ages*, 80.

56　"Indian Cancer Society Inaugurated," *Times of India*, May 3, 1951.

57　"Research Center Opened in Bombay," *Times of India*, December 31, 1952.

58　"Havoc Caused by Cancer in India," *Times of India*, April 5, 1955.

59　"Fight against Cancer," *Times of India*, April 14, 1957; "Treating Cancer," *Times of India*, March 8, 1957.

60　"Cancer Claims 425,000 Lives in India," *Times of India*, January 15, 1969.

61　"Danger of Cancer: India Warned," *Times of India*, April 8, 1970.

62　Sivaramakrishnan, *As the World Ages*, 83.

63　Sivaramakrishnan, *As the World Ages*, 75.

64　Sivaramakrishnan, *As the World Ages*, 84. Indeed, as Sunil Amrith has also argued, the postcolonial state failed to fix the systemic weaknesses of the healthcare system, singling out diseases like malaria or overpopulation for which top-down technical solutions could be proposed. Sunil S. Amrith, *Decolonizing International Health: India and Southeast Asia, 1930–65* (Basingstoke: Palgrave Macmillan, 2006).

65 Madelon Lubin Finkel, *Cancer Screening in the Developing World: Case Studies and Strategies from the Field* (Hanover, NH: Dartmouth College Press, 2018), 6.

66 Charu Bahri, "In an Ominous Sign, India Transits Speedily from Infectious to Lifestyle Diseases," *Scroll.in*, June 10, 2015.

67 Abdel Omran, "The Epidemiologic Transition: A Theory of the Epidemiology of Population Change," *Milbank Memorial Fund Quarterly* 49, no. 4 (1971): 509–38. The theory had languished for two decades after having first been presented in 1971; in recent years, it has been resurrected, reprinted, and widely cited as an explanation for the supposed global explosion of noncommunicable diseases. George Weisz and Jesse Olszynko-Gryn, "The Theory of Epidemiologic Transition: The Origins of a Citation Classic," *Journal of the History of Medicine and Allied Sciences* 65, no. 3 (2010): 287–326.

68 Robin Scheffler points to similar concerns in the United States in the early twentieth century. Robin Wolfe Scheffler, *A Contagious Cause: The American Hunt for Cancer Viruses and the Rise of Molecular Medicine* (Chicago: University of Chicago Press, 2019), 5–7, 251.

69 Lawrence Cohen, *No Aging in India: Alzheimer's, the Bad Family, and Other Modern Things* (Berkeley: University of California Press, 1998).

70 Cohen, *No Aging in India*, 89.

71 Harris Solomon, *Metabolic Living: Food, Fat, and the Absorption of Illness in India* (Durham, NC: Duke University Press, 2016).

72 A leading study found the distribution of cancer prevalence as 110 in 100,000 in urban areas versus 71 in 100,000 in rural areas. Sunil Rajpal, Abhishek Kumar, and William Joe, "Economic Burden of Cancer in India: Evidence from Cross-Sectional Nationally Representative Household Survey, 2014," *PloS One* 13, no. 2 (2018): 1–17.

73 As families are forced to spend about half of the per capita annual household expenditure on cancer hospitalization. Rajpal, Kumar, and Joe, "Economic Burden of Cancer in India."

74 Anshul Kastor and Sanjay K. Mohanty, "Disease-Specific Out-of-Pocket and Catastrophic Health Expenditure on Hospitalization in India: Do Indian Households Face Distress Health Financing?," *PLoS One* 13, no. 5 (2018): e0196106.

75 "Cancerous Trend," *Economic and Political Weekly* 32, no. 24 (1997): 1369.

76 Yashodhara Dalmia, "The Fight against Cancer," *Times of India*, April 20, 1980.

77 Fernandes Allwyn and Mehra Preethi, "Our Hospitals Are Sick," *Times of India*, August 24, 1986.

78 Jain, *Malignant*, 66–67.

79 National Institute of Cancer Prevention and Research, ed., "Dos and Dont's" (Delhi: ICMR, 2019).

80 Cherian Varghese, "Cancer Prevention and Control in India," in *50 Years of Cancer Control in India*, ed. Indian Department of Health (New Delhi: Indian Department of Health, 2003), 48–59.

81 K. Srinath Reddy, Bela Shah, Cherian Varghese, and Anbumani Ramadoss,

"Responding to the Threat of Chronic Diseases in India," *Lancet* 366, no. 9498 (2005): 1744–49.

82 Rajiv Sarin, "Indian National Cancer Control Programme: Setting Sight on Shifting Targets," *Journal of Cancer Research and Therapeutics* 1, no. 4 (2005): 240–48. Another set of researchers helpfully present a proposal to aid the NCCP in setting up basic treatment infrastructures outside urban areas, increasing access to relatively easier-to-deliver chemotherapies and targeted drugs at district level public hospitals S. Gulia, M. Sengar, R. Badwe, and S. Gupta, "National Cancer Control Programme in India: Proposal for Organization of Chemotherapy and Systemic Therapy Services," *Journal of Global Oncology* 3, no. 3 (2017): 271–74. Implicitly, their proposed blueprint shows up the NCCP's long-standing absence of commitment to expanding access to cancer treatments.

83 In her ethnography of cancer in Botswana, Julie Livingston finds similar claims of cancer as a disease of rapid development and finds such claims to be at odds with her ethnographic realities. She shows how epidemiological models dominated by molecular research in the United States obscured the environmental and viral etiologies of the disease, making "African cancers" a conceptual impossibility. Her book goes on to describe the work of improvisation in a cancer ward that is the result of this historical failure, where technologies are either absent or constantly under repair. Livingston, *Improvising Medicine*, 35.

84 Faye Ginsburg, "Culture/Media: A (Mild) Polemic," *Anthropology Today* 10, no. 2 (1994): 13.

85 My aim here is to take Clifford Geertz's simple but difficult insight seriously: "Societies, like lives, contain their own interpretations. One has only to learn how to gain access to them." Clifford Geertz, "Deep Play: Notes on the Balinese Cockfight," in *Interpretation of Cultures* (New York: Basic Books, 1973), 86.

86 Sontag, *Illness as Metaphor*, 3.

87 Susan Sontag, *AIDS and Its Metaphors* (New York: Farrar, Straus and Giroux, 1989), 5.

88 For instance, war metaphors had rationalized the unnecessary suffering and mutilation of a generation of cancer patients as inevitable collateral damage. And the pervasive myth that cancer was brought on by the patient's own depressive personality had stigmatized many others.

89 Ann Jurecic, *Illness as Narrative* (Pittsburgh: University of Pittsburgh Press, 2012), 3–17.

90 So much so that Virginia Woolf bemoaned that "English, which can express the thoughts of Hamlet and the tragedy of Lear, has no words for the shiver and the headache." Virginia Woolf, *On Being Ill* (Paris: Paris Press, 2001), 6.

91 A. H. Hawkins, "Pathography: Patient Narratives of Illness," *Western Journal of Medicine* 171, no. 2 (1999): 127.

92 Jain, *Malignant*.

93 Jain recognizes this too, as she draws upon powerful aesthetic accounts that contest generic trends toward restitution and abstraction.

94 Jurecic, *Illness as Narrative*, 3.

95 Juliet McMullin, "Cancer and the Comics: Graphic Narratives and Biolegitimate Lives," *Medical Anthropology Quarterly* 30, no. 2 (2016): 149–50.

96 Emily Martin, *Bipolar Expeditions: Mania and Depression in American Culture* (Princeton, NJ: Princeton University Press, 2007), 82.

97 The 2015–16 national budget allocated about US$5 billion to health. "Budget Allocation for AIIMS Cut Marginally," *Business Standard*, February 28, 2015.

98 All India Institute of Medical Sciences, "61st AIIMS Annual Report, 2016–2017" (Delhi: AIIMS, 2017).

1. CONCEALING CANCER

1 Mark Davis and Lenore Manderson, *Disclosure in Health and Illness* (London: Routledge, 2014), 15.

2 Davis and Manderson, *Disclosure in Health and Illness*, 155–57.

3 See, for example, Mahati Chittem, Paul Norman, and Peter R. Harris, "Relationships between Perceived Diagnostic Disclosure, Patient Characteristics, Psychological Distress and Illness Perceptions in Indian Cancer Patients," *Psycho-Oncology* 22, no. 6 (2013): 1375–80.

4 Mary-Jo DelVecchio Good, Byron J. Good, Cynthia Schaffer, and Stuart E. Lind, "American Oncology and the Discourse on Hope," *Culture, Medicine and Psychiatry* 14, no. 1 (1990): 59–79; S. E. Lind et al., "Telling the Diagnosis of Cancer," *Journal of Clinical Oncology* 7, no. 5 (1989): 583–89.

5 Cecilia Van Hollen, "Handle with Care: Rethinking the Rights versus Culture Dichotomy in Cancer Disclosure in India," *Medical Anthropology Quarterly* 32, no. 1 (2018): 59–84.

6 Julie Livingston, *Improvising Medicine: An African Oncology Ward in an Emerging Cancer Epidemic* (Durham, NC: Duke University Press, 2012), 166.

7 Harmala Gupta, "A Journey from Cancer to 'Cansupport,'" *Indian Journal of Palliative Care* 10, no. 1 (2004): 32–38.

8 Alyssa Yeager et al., "Cansupport: A Model for Home-Based Palliative Care Delivery in India," *Annals of Palliative Medicine* 5, no. 3 (2016): 166–71.

9 Cecilia Van Hollen, "Nationalism, Transnationalism, and the Politics of 'Traditional' Indian Medicine for HIV/AIDS," in *Asian Medicine and Globalization*, ed. Joseph S. Alter (Philadelphia: University of Pennsylvania Press, 2005), 88–106.

10 Bharat Venkat, "Cures," *Public Culture* 28, no. 3 (80) (2016): 475–97.

11 Byron J. Good et al., "In the Subjunctive Mode: Epilepsy Narratives in Turkey," *Social Science and Medicine* 38, no. 6 (1994): 835–42.

12 Georg Simmel, "The Sociology of Secrecy and of Secret Societies," *American Journal of Sociology* 11, no. 4 (1906): 441–98.

13 Good et al., "In the Subjunctive Mode," 184.

14 For example, L. Nyblade, M. Stockton, S. Travasso, and S. Krishnan, "A Qualitative Exploration of Cervical and Breast Cancer Stigma in Karnataka, India," *BMC Womens Health* 17, no. 1 (2017): 1–15.

15 Such an understanding is closer to Erving Goffman's canonical definition of stigma as contextual and relational and not a direct or predictable outcome of a particular attribute: that is, an attribute that stigmatizes one person might not similarly affect another. Erving Goffman, *Stigma: Notes on the Management of Spoiled Identity* (New York: J. Aronson, 1974), 3. However, I find that the word "stigma" tends to overdetermine the social field in which the practices of nondisclosure appear. Rather than try to recover it, I try here to think outside the concept of stigma to open more careful descriptions of the relation between nondisclosure and everyday life.

16 My thanks to the second press reader for helping me clarify this formulation.

17 Dwaipayan Banerjee, "Markets and Molecules: A Pharmaceutical Primer from the South," *Medical Anthropology* 36, no. 4 (2017): 363–80.

18 Stefan Ecks, "Global Pharmaceutical Markets and Corporate Citizenship: The Case of Novartis' Anti-cancer Drug Glivec," *BioSocieties* 3 (2008): 165–81.

19 Alex Broom and Assa Doron, "The Rise of Cancer in Urban India: Cultural Understandings, Structural Inequalities and the Emergence of the Clinic," *Health* 16, no. 3 (2012): 250–66.

20 Veena Das, *Affliction: Health, Disease, Poverty* (New York: Fordham University Press, 2015).

21 Sarah Pinto, *Where There Is No Midwife: Birth and Loss in Rural India* (New York: Berghahn Books, 2008).

22 As Holly Donahue Singh describes in her analysis of fertility treatment in North India, strategies of disclosure and nondisclosure are never straightforward evidence of either liberation or autonomy but are enmeshed with the structures of everyday life and kinship. Holly Donahue Singh, "Fertility Control: Reproductive Desires, Kin Work, and Women's Status in Contemporary India," *Medical Anthropology Quarterly* 31, no. 1 (2017): 23–39.

23 Tom Boellstorff, "Nuri's Testimony: HIV/AIDS in Indonesia and Bare Knowledge," *American Ethnologist* 36, no. 2 (2009): 356.

24 Kate Wood and Helen Lambert, "Coded Talk, Scripted Omissions," *Medical Anthropology Quarterly* 22, no. 3 (2008): 213–33.

25 Wood and Lambert, "Coded Talk, Scripted Omissions," 215.

26 Wood and Lambert, "Coded Talk, Scripted Omissions," 216.

27 Mathew Sunil George and Helen Lambert, "'I Am Doing Fine Only Because I Have Not Told Anyone': The Necessity of Concealment in the Lives of People Living with HIV in India," *Culture, Health and Sexuality* 17, no. 8 (2015): 933–46.

28 Adam Seligman, Robert Weller, Michael Puett, and Bennett Simon, *Ritual and Its Consequences: An Essay on the Limits of Sincerity* (Oxford: Oxford University Press, 2008); Vaibhav Saria, "To Be Some Other Name: The Naming Games That Hijras Play," *South Asia Multidisciplinary Academic Journal*, no. 12 (2015): 1–16.

29 Fiona Graham and David Clark, "Definition and Evaluation: Developing the Debate on Community Participation in Palliative Care," *Indian Journal of Palliative Care* 11, no. 1 (2005): 2–5.

30   Suresh Kumar and Mathews Numpeli, "Neighborhood Network in Palliative Care," *Indian Journal of Palliative Care* 11, no. 1 (2005): 6–9.

31   Harmala Gupta, "Community Participation in Palliative Care: A Comment," *Indian Journal of Palliative Care* 11, no. 1 (2005): 19.

32   Gupta, "Community Participation in Palliative Care," 21.

33   Jan Stjernswärd, "Community Participation in Palliative Care," *Indian Journal of Palliative Care* 11, no. 1 (2005): 27.

34   For an overview of the history of community participation, see Lynn M. Morgan, "Community Participation in Health: Perpetual Allure, Persistent Challenge," *Health Policy and Planning* 16, no. 3 (2001): 221–30; Susan B. Rifkin, "Paradigms Lost: Toward a New Understanding of Community Participation in Health Programmes," *Acta Tropica* 61, no. 2 (1996): 79–92.

35   Madan, like many other public health scholars, expressed disappointment about how the idea of community participation has played out in practice. He pointed out that the idea of participation did not address the power inequality between governments and citizens. Further, he argues, the undifferentiated idea of "community" romanticized the poor, ignoring the complex nature of hierarchies that divide every social collective. T. N. Madan, "Community Involvement in Health Policy: Socio-structural and Dynamic Aspects of Health Beliefs," *Social Science and Medicine* 25, no. 6 (1987): 615–20.

36   As Smarajit Jana writes in the context of sex-work organization around the HIV-AIDS crisis in Bengal, this discourse of community empowerment raised many challenges. In her experience, "community mobilization" erroneously imagined that there was a stable, cooperative constituency of sex workers waiting to be brought into social action. Smarajit Jana, "Community Mobilisation: Myths and Challenges," *Journal of Epidemiology and Community Health* 66, no. 2 (2012): ii5–ii6.

37   For an overview written by key drafters of the process, see Thomas Isaac and Richard Franke, *Local Democracy and Development: The Kerala People's Campaign for Decentralized Planning* (Lanham, MD: Rowman and Littlefield, 2002).

38   Rama V. Baru et al., "Inequities in Access to Health Services in India: Caste, Class and Region," *Economic and Political Weekly* 45, no. 38 (2010): 49–58; C. U. Thresia, "Rising Private Sector and Falling 'Good Health at Low Cost': Health Challenges in China, Sri Lanka, and Indian State of Kerala," *International Journal of Health Services* 43, no. 1 (2013): 31–48.

39   Elizabeth McDermott, Lucy Selman, Michael Wright, and David Clark, "Hospice and Palliative Care Development in India: A Multimethod Review of Services and Experiences," *Journal of Pain and Symptom Management* 35, no. 6 (2008): 583–93.

40   For more on a South Asian social reformist template for establishing ties through, as well as beyond, blood, see Jacob Copeman and Dwaipayan Banerjee, *Hematologies: The Political Life of Blood in India* (Ithaca, NY: Cornell University Press, 2019), 88–92.

41   Pinto, *Where There Is No Midwife*.

42 Lawrence Martis and Anne Westhues, "A Synthesis of the Literature on Breaking Bad News or Truth Telling: Potential for Research in India," *Indian Journal of Palliative Care* 19, no. 1 (2013): 2–11.

43 For example, Santosh K. Chaturvedi, Carmen G. Loiselle, and Prabha S. Chandra, "Communication with Relatives and Collusion in Palliative Care: A Cross-Cultural Perspective," *Indian Journal of Palliative Care* 15, no. 1 (2009): 2–9.

44 For example, P. John Alexander, Narayanakurup Dinesh, and M. S. Vidyasagar, "Psychiatric Morbidity among Cancer Patients and Its Relationship with Awareness of Illness and Expectations about Treatment Outcome," *Acta Oncologica* 32, no. 6 (1993): 623–26; Prabha S. Chandra et al., "Awareness of Diagnosis and Psychiatric Morbidity among Cancer Patients: A Study from South India," *Journal of Psychosomatic Research* 45, no. 3 (1998): 257–61.

45 For example, D. Purakkal, D. Pulassery, and S. Ravindran, "Should a Patient with a Life Threatening Illness Be Informed of the Diagnosis? A Survey of Physicians and Medical Students in Calicut," *Indian Journal of Palliative Care* 10, no. 2 (2004): 64–66.

46 For example, Prabha S. Chandra and Geetha Desai, "Denial as an Experiential Phenomenon in Serious Illness," *Indian Journal of Palliative Care* 13, no. 1 (2007): 8–14.

2. CANCER CONJUGALITY

1 Alyssa Yeager et al., "Cansupport: A Model for Home-Based Palliative Care Delivery in India," *Annals of Palliative Medicine* 5, no. 3 (2016): 168; S. Lukhmana, S. Bhasin, P. Chhabra, and M. Bhatia, "Family Caregivers' Burden: A Hospital Based Study in 2010 among Cancer Patients from Delhi," *Indian Journal of Cancer* 52, no. 1 (2015): 148.

2 Shalini Grover, *Marriage, Love, Caste, and Kinship Support: Lived Experiences of the Urban Poor in India* (New Delhi: Social Science Press, 2011); Saraswati Haider, "Migrant Women and Urban Experience in a Squatter Settlement," in *Delhi: Urban Space and Human Destinies*, ed. Veronique Dupont, Emma Tarlo, and Denis Vidal (New Delhi: Manohar, 2000), 29–49.

3 Claire Natalie Snell-Rood, *No One Will Let Her Live: Women's Struggle for Well-Being in a Delhi Slum* (Oakland: University of California Press, 2015), 3.

4 Veena Das and Ranendra Kumar Das, *The Interface between Mental Health and Reproductive Health of Women among the Urban Poor in Delhi* (Thiruvananthapuram: Achutha Menon Centre for Health Science Studies, Sree Chitra Tirunal Institute for Medical Sciences and Technology, 2005), 36; Kumkum Sangari, "Violent Acts: Cultures, Structures and Retraditionalisation," in *Women of India: Colonial and Post-colonial Periods*, ed. Bharati Ray (Delhi: Sage, 2005), 159–81.

5 See, for some examples, Katherine Lemons, "The Politics of Livability: Tutoring 'Kinwork' in a New Delhi Women's Arbitration Center," *PoLAR: Political and Legal Anthropology Review* 39, no. 2 (2016): 244–60; Julia Kowalski, "Ordering Dependence: Care, Disorder, and Kinship Ideology in North Indian Antivio-

lence Counseling," *American Ethnologist* 43, no. 1 (2016): 63–75; Srimati Basu, "Judges of Normality: Mediating Marriage in the Family Courts of Kolkata, India," *Signs: Journal of Women in Culture and Society* 37, no. 2 (2012): 469–92; Sylvia Vatuk, "The 'Women's Court' in India: An Alternative Dispute Resolution Body for Women in Distress," *Journal of Legal Pluralism and Unofficial Law* 45, no. 1 (2013): 76–103. See also Amita Singh and Patricia Uberoi's work describing a similar tendency toward advising acceptance and reconciliation in women's popular fiction. Amita Tyagi Singh and Patricia Uberoi, "Learning to 'Adjust': Conjugal Relations in Indian Popular Fiction," *Bulletin (Centre for Women's Development Studies)* 1, no. 1 (1994): 93–120.

6 Rajni Palriwala and Ravinder Kaur, "Marriage in South Asia: Continuities and Transformations," in *Marrying in South Asia: Shifting Concepts, Changing Practices in a Globalizing World*, ed. Rajni Palriwala and Ravinder Kaur (Delhi: Orient Blackswan, 2014), 21.

7 Elizabeth A. Povinelli, *The Empire of Love: Toward a Theory of Intimacy, Genealogy, and Carnality* (Durham, NC: Duke University Press, 2006), 6.

8 Flavia Agnes, "The Supreme Court, the Media, and the Uniform Civil Code Debate in India," in *The Crisis of Secularism in India*, ed. Anuradha Dingwaney Needham and Rajeswari Sunder Rajan (Durham, NC: Duke University Press, 2007), 294–315.

9 Clara Han, *Life in Debt: Times of Care and Violence in Neoliberal Chile* (Berkeley: University of California Press, 2012), 5.

10 Zoë H. Wool, *After War: The Weight of Life at Walter Reed* (Durham, NC: Duke University Press, 2015), 22; Veena Das, *Affliction: Health, Disease, Poverty* (New York: Fordham University Press, 2015), 26.

11 Crimes such as these that come under the legal category of "crimes of honor" have attracted much public and scholarly attention. For a conceptualization of this phenomenon as crimes against women and the problems with the public framing of "honor killings," see Uma Chakravarti, "From Fathers to Husbands: Of Love, Death and Marriage in North India," in *Honour Crimes, Paradigms, and Violence against Women*, ed. Lynn Welcgan and Sarah Hossain (London: Zed Books, 2005), 309.

12 In another context, Pocock highlights the difficulties of translating the concept of sevā, as it moves across theology and personal relations. The possibilities range from "devotion" to "intimate care." Here, I translate it simply as "care," leaving it flexible enough to lend itself to multiple interpretations. D. F. Pocock, "Preservation of the Religious Life: Hindu Immigrants in England," *Contributions to Indian Sociology* 10, no. 2 (1976): 341–65.

13 Lawrence Cohen, *No Aging in India: Alzheimer's, the Bad Family, and Other Modern Things* (Berkeley: University of California Press, 1998), 57–61; Sarah Lamb, *White Saris and Sweet Mangoes: Aging, Gender, and Body in North India* (Berkeley: University of California Press, 2000).

14 Kowalski, "Ordering Dependence," 64.

15 Sarah Pinto, *The Doctor and Mrs. A.: Ethics and Counter-ethics in an Indian Dream Analysis* (New York: Fordham University Press, 2019).

16 Veena Das, "What Does Ordinary Ethics Look Like?," in *Four Lectures on Ethics*, ed. Michael Lambek, Veena Das, Didier Fassin, and Webb Keane (Chicago: HAU Books, 2015), 116.

17 Michael M. J. Fischer, "Urban Mahabharata: Health Care, Ordinary, Traditional, and Contemporary Ethics," *Medicine Anthropology Theory* 4, no. 3 (2017): 98–129.

18 For the purposes of clarity, I will minimize the number of times I cite Pinto's influence in the following paragraphs, but I want to make clear that I depend on her prior reading of every mythic figure that I invoke here. Pinto, *The Doctor and Mrs. A.*

19 Pinto, *The Doctor and Mrs. A.*

20 Veena Das, *Life and Words: Violence and the Descent into the Ordinary* (Berkeley: University of California Press, 2007), 104, 216.

21. Veena Das, "Violence and Nonviolence at the Heart of Hindu Ethics," in *The Oxford Handbook of Religion and Violence*, ed. Michael Jerryson, Mark Juergensmeyer, and Margo Kitts (Oxford: Oxford University Press, 2013), 26–27. See also Das, "War and the Mythological Imagination," *Antropologia*, no. 16 (2013): 25–35.

22 See, for one canonical reading Judith Butler, *Antigone's Claim: Kinship between Life and Death* (New York: Columbia University Press, 2000).

3. RESEARCHING PAIN, PRACTICING EMPATHY

1 D. Hui et al., "Availability and Integration of Palliative Care at US Cancer Centers," *JAMA* 303, no. 11 (2010): 1054–61. A more recent study by the National Cancer Institute–recognized comprehensive cancer care centers in the United States still had the number at less than one-third. Sheila L. Hammer, Karen Clark, Marcia Grant, and Matthew J. Loscalzo, "Seventeen Years of Progress for Supportive Care Services: A Resurvey of National Cancer Institute–Designated Comprehensive Cancer Centers," *Palliative and Supportive Care* 13, no. 4 (2015): 917–25.

2 Thomas Lynch, Stephen Connor, and David Clark, "Mapping Levels of Palliative Care Development: A Global Update," *Journal of Pain and Symptom Management* 45, no. 6 (2013): 1094–106.

3 "Budget Allocation for AIIMS Cut Marginally," *Business Standard*, February 28, 2015.

4 Susan W. Hinze, "Gender and the Body of Medicine or at Least Some Body Parts: (Re)Constructing the Prestige Hierarchy of Medical Specialties," *Sociological Quarterly* 40, no. 2 (1999): 217–39.

5 Sarah Pinto, *Daughters of Parvati: Women and Madness in Contemporary India* (Philadelphia: University of Pennsylvania Press, 2014), 56; Cecilia Van Hollen, *Birth on the Threshold: Childbirth and Modernity in South India* (Berkeley: University of California Press, 2003), 127. Further, even those with the most

progressive ambitions for the field do not ask that anesthesiologists play a role in public health beyond aiding surgery and perioperative care. See, for example, Ram Roth, Elizabeth A. M. Frost, Clifford Gevirtz, and Carrie L. H. Atcheson, *The Role of Anesthesiology in Global Health: A Comprehensive Guide* (New York: Springer, 2015).

6 Ajantha Subramanian, "Making Merit: The Indian Institutes of Technology and the Social Life of Caste," *Comparative Studies in Society and History* 57, no. 2 (2015): 291–322.

7 Srirupa Roy, *Beyond Belief: India and the Politics of Postcolonial Nationalism* (Durham, NC: Duke University Press, 2007).

8 Archibald Vivian Hill, "A Report to the Government of India on Scientific Research in India" (London: Royal Society, 1945).

9 Joseph Bhore, "Report of the Health Survey and Development Committee. Vol. 2. Recommendations" (Delhi: Government of India, 1946).

10 For her dissertation on medical education at AIIMS, Anna Ruddock interviewed several doctors who joined the institute at its inception. Each of these doctors recollected that they had joined the institute as researchers; they had been told that its function as a referral hospital for tertiary care was secondary to its scientific ambitions. Yet, unable to keep the outside at bay, in the decades since its founding AIIMS has steadily grown into one of the largest general hospitals in the world. Anna Louise Ruddock, "Special Medicine: Producing Doctors at the All India Institute of Medical Sciences (AIIMS)" (PhD diss., King's College London, 2017).

11 I am thinking here of ruin in the sense of Ann Stoler's formulation of the term as verb and noun. Here, the ruin codes a layering of historical operations of colonial and postcolonial power. If Nehru's vision is indebted in part to an Enlightenment project of scientific rationality, in the present AIIMS continues to carry this historic promise of scientific purity and rational governance. In the present, contemporary caste politics, political economic transformations, and forms of particular identity continuously challenge this embattled promise. Ann Laura Stoler, "Imperial Debris: Reflections on Ruins and Ruination," *Cultural Anthropology* 23, no. 2 (2008): 191–219.

12 Julie Livingston, *Improvising Medicine: An African Oncology Ward in an Emerging Cancer Epidemic* (Durham, DC: Duke University Press, 2012).

13 Kounteya Sinha, "Even a CAT Scan Has a 4-Month Wait List at AIIMS," *Times of India*, October 9, 2011.

14 Marieke H. J. van den Beuken–van Everdingen et al., "Update on Prevalence of Pain in Patients with Cancer: Systematic Review and Meta-analysis," *Journal of Pain and Symptom Management* 51, no. 6 (2016): 1070–90.

15 Felicia Marie Knaul et al., "Alleviating the Access Abyss in Palliative Care and Pain Relief—an Imperative of Universal Health Coverage: The Lancet Commission Report," *Lancet* 391, no. 10128 (2018): 1391–454.

16 The only countries in this category outside the United States and Europe were Australia, Hong Kong, Japan, Singapore, and Uganda.

17 To preserve anonymity, I have changed the names of all AIIMS researchers and physicians. In this chapter, I have retained the original names only of researchers at other institutions whose work I quote as secondary, published sources.

18 Tim Wigmore, Vijaya Gottumukkala, and Bernhard Riedel, "Making the Case for the Subspecialty of Onco-Anesthesia," *International Anesthesiology Clinics* 54, no. 4 (2016): 19–28.

19 Reference withheld to preserve anonymity.

20 Reference withheld to preserve anonymity.

21 B. Thomas, Manoj Pandey, K. Ramdas, and Muthu Nair, "Psychological Distress in Cancer Patients: Hypothesis of a Distress Model," *European Journal of Cancer Prevention* 11, no. 2 (2002): 179–85.

22 Michael Polanyi, *The Tacit Dimension* (London: Routledge, 1967).

23 James Mill, *The History of British India* (London: Printed for Baldwin, Cradock, and Joy, 1817); F. Max Muller, *India, What Can It Teach Us? A Course of Lectures* (London: Longmans, Green, 1883); Max Weber, *The Religion of India: The Sociology of Hinduism and Buddhism* (Glencoe, IL: Free Press, 1958).

24 M. B. Singer, *When a Great Tradition Modernizes* (Chicago: University of Chicago Press, 1972); James Laidlaw, "For an Anthropology of Ethics and Freedom," *Journal of the Royal Anthropological Institute* 8, no. 2 (2002): 311–32; Nicholas B. Dirks, *Castes of Mind: Colonialism and the Making of Modern India* (Princeton, NJ: Princeton University Press, 2001).

25 S. Cromwell Crawford, *The Evolution of Hindu Ethical Ideals* (Manoa: University of Hawaii Press, 1974); Crawford, *Dilemmas of Life and Death: Hindu Ethics in North American Context* (Albany, NY: SUNY Press, 1995); Crawford, *Hindu Bioethics for the Twenty-First Century* (Albany, NY: SUNY Press, 2003); S. Firth, "End-of-Life:
A Hindu View," *Lancet* 366, no. 9486 (2005): 682–86.

26 C. Laubry and T. Brosse, "Data Gathered in India on a Yogi with Simultaneous Registration of the Pulse, Respiration, and Electrocardiogram," *Presse Medicale* 44 (1936): 1601–4.

27 M. A. Wenger, B. K. Bagchi, and B. K. Anand, "Experiments in India on 'Voluntary' Control of the Heart and Pulse," *Circulation* 24, no. 6 (1961): 1319–25.

28 B. K. Anand, G. S. Chinna, and B. Singh, "Studies on Shri Ramanand Yogi during His Stay in an Air-Tight Box," *Indian Journal of Medical Research* 49, no. 1 (1961): 82–89.

29 William J. Broad, *The Science of Yoga: The Risks and the Rewards* (New York: Simon and Schuster, 2012).

30 Projit Bihari Mukharji, *Doctoring Traditions: Ayurveda, Small Technologies, and Braided Sciences* (Chicago: University of Chicago Press, 2016).

31 Subhash Kirpekar, "Science and Yoga," *Times of India*, June 29, 1969.

32 Pamela Jeter, Jerry Slutsky, Nilkamal Singh, and Sat Bir Khalsa, "Yoga as a Therapeutic Intervention: A Bibliometric Analysis of Published Research Studies from 1967 to 2013," *Journal of Alternative and Complementary Medicine* 21, no. 10 (2015): 586–92.

33 Neena Kohli and Ajit K. Dalal, "Culture as a Factor in Causal Understanding of Illness: A Study of Cancer Patients," *Psychology and Developing Societies* 10, no. 2 (1998): 115–29.

34 Ajit K. Dalal, "Living with a Chronic Disease: Healing and Psychological Adjustment in Indian Society," *Psychology and Developing Societies* 12, no. 1 (2000): 67–81.

35 S. Vasudevan, "Coping with Terminal Illness: A Spiritual Perspective," *Indian Journal of Palliative Care* 9, no. 1 (2003): 19.

36 Kohli and Dalal, "Culture as a Factor in Causal Understanding of Illness."

37 Prabha S. Chandra et al., "Awareness of Diagnosis and Psychiatric Morbidity among Cancer Patients: A Study from South India," *Journal of Psychosomatic Research* 45, no. 3 (1998): 257–61; Santosh K. Chaturvedi, "Ethical Dilemmas in Palliative Care in Traditional Developing Societies, with Special Reference to the Indian Setting," *Journal of Medical Ethics* 34, no. 8 (2008): 611–15; Chaturvedi, "Spiritual Issues at End of Life," *Indian Journal of Palliative Care* 13, no. 2 (2007): 48; Chaturvedi, "What's Important for Quality of Life to Indians—in Relation to Cancer," *Social Science and Medicine* 33, no. 1 (1991): 91–94; Santosh K. Chaturvedi, Carmen G. Loiselle, and Prabha S. Chandra, "Communication with Relatives and Collusion in Palliative Care: A Cross-Cultural Perspective," *Indian Journal of Palliative Care* 15, no. 1 (2009): 2–9; A. Kandasamy, S. K. Chaturvedi, and G. Desai, "Spirituality, Distress, Depression, Anxiety, and Quality of Life in Patients with Advanced Cancer," *Indian Journal of Cancer* 48, no. 1 (2011): 55–59.

38 Reference withheld to preserve anonymity.

39 Tulasi Srinivas, "Artful Living," in *Critical Themes in Indian Sociology*, ed. Sanjay Srivastava, Yasmeen Arif, and Janaki Abraham (New Delhi: Sage, 2018), 62–76.

40 Joanne Punzo Waghorne, "Engineering an Artful Practice: On Jaggi Vasudev's Isha Yoga and Sri Sri Ravishankar's Art of Living," in *Gurus of Modern Yoga*, ed. Mark Singleton and Ellen Goldberg (New York: Oxford University Press, 2013), 283–307.

41 Nandini Gooptu, "New Spirituality, Politics of Self-Empowerment, Citizenship, and Democracy in Contemporary India," *Modern Asian Studies* 50, no. 3 (2016): 934–74.

42 During my fieldwork, the health care rights NGO Swasthya Adhikar Manch filed a public interest litigation in the Supreme Court. In 2013, the Court responded with a harsh indictment of the government, citing that at least 2,374 people had died as a result of ethically dubious trials in the period between 2007 and 2012.

43 Kaushik Sunder Rajan, "The Experimental Machinery of Global Clinical Trials: Case Studies from India," *Asian Biotech* 38, no. 1 (2010): 55–80.

44 It is worth noting, however, that about three-quarters of the subjects were literate, and more than half the patients lived in the city, a slight departure from the usual demographic pattern of patients at AIIMS.

45 Reference withheld to preserve anonymity.

46 Rajkumari Tankha, "Reason the Centre for Integrative Medicine and Research at AIIMS Is a Boon," *Narada News*, June 2016, http://naradanews.com/2016/06/reason-the-centre-for-integrative-medicine-and-research-at-aiims-is-a-boon/.

47 "AIIMS Gets New Centre for Integrative Medicine and Research (CIMR)," *Medical Dialogues: Voices of the Medical Profession*, June 23, 2016, https://medical dialogues.in/aiims-gets-new-centre-for-integrative-medicine-and-research-cimr/.

48 Helena Hansen and Mary E. Skinner, "From White Bullets to Black Markets and Greened Medicine: The Neuroeconomics and Neuroracial Politics of Opioid Pharmaceuticals," *Annals of Anthropological Practice* 36, no. 1 (2012): 167–82.

49 The research on the patterns of addiction relating to oral morphine consumption in North India is still inconclusive. A study conducted by the Department of Psychiatry at AIIMS found high levels of opioid addiction, but it also found that the form most frequently abused was heroin. Yatan Pal Singh Balhara, Rajeev Ranjan, Anju Dhawan, and Deepak Yadav, "Experiences from a Community Based Substance Use Treatment Centre in an Urban Resettlement Colony in India," *Journal of Addiction* 2014 (2014): 1–6. In contrast, however, another study conducted by the department with a smaller sample of thirty-one patients found that among women, abuse of prescriptions for pain relief was actually quite common. Prabhoo Dayal and Yatan Pal Singh Balhara, "Profile of Female Patients Seeking In-Patient Treatment for Prescription Opioid Abuse from a Tertiary Care Drug Dependence Treatment Centre from India," *Indian Journal of Medical Research* 143, no. 1 (2016): 95–100.

50 M. R. Rajagopal and David E. Joranson, "India: Opioid Availability; an Update," *Journal of Pain and Symptom Management* 33, no. 5 (2007): 615–22.

51 Elaine Scarry's description of this problem of pain is both canonical and its most extreme formulation. Elaine Scarry, *The Body in Pain: The Making and Unmaking of the World* (New York: Oxford University Press, 1985).

52 Ronald Melzack and Patrick Wall, "Pain Mechanisms: A New Theory," *Science* 150, no. 3699 (1965): 971–79.

53 Ronald Melzack, "Phantom Limbs and the Concept of a Neuromatrix," *Trends in Neurosciences* 13, no. 3 (1990): 88–92.

54 Ronald Melzack, "Phantom Limbs," *Scientific American*, September 1, 2006, https://www.scientificamerican.com/article/phantom-limbs-2006-09/.

55 T. Anand et al., "Workplace Violence against Resident Doctors in a Tertiary Care Hospital in Delhi," *National Medical Journal of India* 29, no. 6 (2016): 344–48.

56 Sumegha Gulati, "The Last Dispatch," *Caravan*, November 30, 2016, https://caravanmagazine.in/essay/last-dispatch-sumegha-gulati-cancer-memoir.

57 Luc Boltanski, *Distant Suffering: Morality, Media and Politics* (Cambridge: Cambridge University Press, 1999).

4. CANCER MEMOIRS

1   Minakshi Chaudhry, *Sunshine: My Encounter with Cancer* (New Delhi: Rupa, 2011), 17.

2   Neelam Kumar, *To Cancer, with Love: My Journey of Joy* (Delhi: Hay House, 2015), 22.

3   Moitreyee Saha, *My Date with Cancer* (Gurgaon: Partridge, 2014), 44–48.

4   Anup Kumar, *The Joy of Cancer* (New Delhi: Rupa, 2002), 29.

5   Mammen Varghese, *Upgraded to Life* (Bangalore: Pothi, 2016), 18; Usha Jesudasan, *Two Journeys: The Challenges of Breast Cancer* (Bengaluru: Berean Bay Media House, 2016).

6   N. Kumar, *To Cancer, with Love*, 64.

7   N. Kumar, *To Cancer, with Love*, 47.

8   N. Kumar, *To Cancer, with Love*, 50.

9   Kamlesh Tripathi, *Gloom behind the Smile* (New Delhi: Pigeon Books, 2012), 137.

10 Vijay Anand Reddy, *I Am a Survivor* (New Delhi: Penguin Random House India, 2017), 123.

11 Roopa Venkatesh, *Cancer: A Comma, Not a Fullstop* (New Delhi: Shroff, 2013), 12.

12 Nitin Unkule, *Cancer Care and Mysteries and Yoga* (Pune, Maharashtra: Mehta, 2010).

13 For a review of this trope in Europe and the United States, see H. J. Eysenck, "Cancer, Personality and Stress: Prediction and Prevention," *Advances in Behaviour Research and Therapy* 16, no. 3 (1994): 167–215.

14 Lauren Berlant, *The Female Complaint* (Durham, NC: Duke University Press, 2008).

15 Lauren Berlant, *Cruel Optimism* (Durham, NC: Duke University Press, 2011).

16 Kathlyn Conway, *Ordinary Life: A Memoir of Illness* (Ann Arbor: University of Michigan Press, 2007), 1.

17 Kathlyn Conway, *Beyond Words: Illness and the Limits of Expression* (Albuquerque: University of New Mexico Press, 2013), 4; Arthur W. Frank, *The Wounded Storyteller: Body, Illness, and Ethics* (Chicago: University of Chicago Press, 1995); Reynolds Price, *A Whole New Life: An Illness and a Healing* (New York: Scribner, 2003).

18 Price, *A Whole New Life*, 180.

19 Conway, *Ordinary Life*, 2; Conway, *Beyond Words*, 9.

20 Ann Jurecic, *Illness as Narrative* (Pittsburgh: University of Pittsburgh Press, 2012).

21 For recent best sellers that reflect this trend, see Atul Gawande, *Being Mortal: Medicine and What Matters in the End* (New York: Metropolitan Books, 2014); Paul Kalanithi, *When Breath Becomes Air* (New York: Random House, 2016).

22 Gawande, *Being Mortal*, 8.

23 Nazeem Beegum, *My Mother Did Not Go Bald: Memoir of a Daughter* (Kottayam: Expressions, 2014).

24 See, for example, Peter Metcalf and Richard Huntington, *Celebrations of Death:*

The Anthropology of Mortuary Ritual (Cambridge: Cambridge University Press, 1991).

25 Anand Prakash Maheshwari, *Mayan* (Delhi: Prabhat Prakashan, 2012).

26 *Mayan* is not alone in drawing an analogy between the experience of cancer and this episode in the Gita. For example, in his memoir, the journalist Krishna Vattam makes an analogy between the ethical struggle of the cancer patient and Arjuna's quandary. Both, Vattam suggests, are humbled by the prospect of death: while the patient fears his own, Arjuna fears inflicting it on others. And both are compelled by forces outside their control; Arjuna is compelled by his duty as a warrior, and the patient is compelled by disease.

27 Amita Malhotra, *Silent Echoes: A True Story* (New Delhi: New Dawn, 2005), 89.

28 Malhotra, *Silent Echoes*, 117.

29 Malhotra, *Silent Echoes*, 132.

5. CANCER FILMS

1 Sanghamitra Pati, "Bollywood's Cancer: Disconnect between Reel and Real Oncology," *Cancer and Society* 16, no. 8 (2015): 894–95.

2 Harshal Pandve, "Cancer and Indian Films," *Journal of Cancer Research and Therapeutics* 6, no. 2 (2010): 233.

3 Vijay Anand Reddy, *I Am a Survivor* (New Delhi: Penguin Random House India, 2017), 316.

4 Ravi Vasudevan, *The Melodramatic Public: Film Form and Spectatorship in Indian Cinema* (Ranikhet: Permanent Black, 2011); Tejaswini Ganti, "Sentiments of Disdain and Practices of Distinction: Boundary-Work, Subjectivity, and Value in the Hindi Film Industry," *Anthropological Quarterly* 85, no. 1 (2012): 5–43.

5 Madhava Prasad, "Diverting Diseases," in *Figurations in Indian Film*, ed. Anustup Basu and Meheli Sen (London: Palgrave Macmillan, 2013).

6 While the Widow Remarriage Act legalized the practice in 1856, the practice remained common and an area of prominent policy concern for the postcolonial state.

7 Wendy Doniger, *On Hinduism* (Oxford: Oxford University Press, 2014), 523.

8 Linda Williams, "Melodrama Revised," in *Refiguring American Film Genres: History and Theory*, ed. Nick Browne (Berkeley: University of California Press, 1998), 42–88.

9 Peter Brooks, *The Melodramatic Imagination: Balzac, Henry James, Melodrama, and the Mode of Excess* (New Haven, CT: Yale University Press, 1976).

10 Vasudevan, *The Melodramatic Public*, 108.

11 See, for example, Mary Ann Doane, *The Desire to Desire: The Woman's Film of the 1940s* (Bloomington: Indiana University Press, 1987).

12 Christine Gledhill, "The Melodramatic Field: An Investigation," in *Home Is Where the Heart Is: Studies in Melodrama and the Woman's Film*, ed. Christine Gledhill (London: BFI Publishing, 1987). See also Williams, "Melodrama Revised."

13   Ira Bhaskar, "Emotion, Subjectivity, and the Limits of Desire: Melodrama and Modernity in Bombay Cinema, 1940s–'50s," in *Gender Meets Genre in Postwar Cinemas*, ed. Christine Gledhill (Urbana: University of Illinois Press, 2012), 163.

14   Shoma Chatterji, "Hrishikesh Mukherjee: Giving Cinema a New Definition," *Silhouette*, September 30, 2015, https://learningandcreativity.com/silhouette/hrishikesh-mukherjee-interview/.

15   The heroism of Anand as a cancer patient became legendary among film watchers; his diagnosis, "lymphosarcoma of the intestine," is synonymous with the disease for anyone with an interest in Hindi films. For its ubiquity, the diagnosis has also drawn the ire of those demanding realism from cancer films. As one blogger put it, the film elevated a very obscure cancer to the limelight, whereas it could have chosen so many more common cancers to raise awareness about them. Mrs 55, "Lymphosarcoma of the Intestine: The Making of a Bollywood Legend," *Mr. and Mrs. 55—Classic Bollywood Revisited*, https://mrandmrs55.com/2012/02/20/lymphosarcoma-of-the-intestine-the-making-of-a-bollywood-legend/.

16   Lawrence Cohen, "Foreign Operations: Reflections on Clinical Mobility in Indian Film and Beyond," in *Critical Mobilities*, ed. Ola Soderstrom et al. (Abingdon, UK: Routledge, 2013), 213–34.

17   The shifting imagination of the "'foreign operation" is precisely what interests Lawrence Cohen in his description of the staging of class mobility and geography in Hindi film. Cohen, "Foreign Operations."

18   Tejaswini Ganti, *Producing Bollywood: Inside the Contemporary Hindi Film Industry* (Durham, NC: Duke University Press, 2012).

19   See Sudhavna Deshpande, "The Consumable Hero of Globalized India," in *Bollyworld: Popular Indian Cinema through a Transnational Lens*, ed. Raminder Kaur and Ajay Sinha (New Delhi: Sage, 2005).

20   IANS, "Sanjay Dutt Gets Teary Eyed; Recalls Nargis Dutt's Fight against Cancer," DNA India, accessed December 7, 2019, http://www.dnaindia.com/entertainment/report-sanjay-dutt-gets-teary-eyed-recalls-nargis-dutt-s-fight-against-cancer-1771416.

21   I explore the institutional ramifications of this incident in chapter 1, as it catalyzed the foundation of AIIMS.

22   Padmakar Darne, "Misconceptions about Cancer Therapy," *Economic and Political Weekly* 12, no. 44 (1977): 1844–45.

23   Cohen, "Foreign Operations," 231–33.

24   Kathlyn Conway, *Beyond Words: Illness and the Limits of Expression* (Albuquerque: University of New Mexico Press, 2013), 16.

6. ENDURANCE

Epigraph: Zoë H. Wool, "In-Durable Sociality: Precarious Life in Common and the Temporal Boundaries of the Social," *Social Text* 35, no. 1 (130) (2017): 80.

1 Joel Robbins, "Beyond the Suffering Subject: Toward an Anthropology of the Good," *Journal of the Royal Anthropological Institute* 19, no. 3 (2013): 447–62; Harry Walker and Iza Kavedžija, "Values of Happiness," *HAU: Journal of Ethnographic Theory* 5, no. 3 (2015): 1–23. For discussions of this critique, see Sherry B. Ortner, "Dark Anthropology and Its Others," *HAU: Journal of Ethnographic Theory* 6, no. 1 (2016): 47–73; Bruce Knauft, "Good Anthropology in Dark Times: Critical Appraisal and Ethnographic Application," *Australian Journal of Anthropology* 30 (2018): 3–17; Miriam Ticktin, "Transnational Humanitarianism," *Annual Review of Anthropology* 43, no. 1 (2014): 273–89.

2 Robbins, "Beyond the Suffering Subject," 448.

3 Tobias Kelly, "A Life Less Miserable?," *HAU: Journal of Ethnographic Theory* 3, no. 1 (2013): 213–16. One answer, Don Kulick suggests, is as compelling as it is troubling: that anthropologists derive a masochistic pleasure from identifications with the powerless. Don Kulick, "Theory in Furs: Masochist Anthropology," *Current Anthropology* 47, no. 6 (2006): 933–52.

4 For a discussion of the ethics of journalistic representations of health suffering, see Arthur Kleinman and Joan Kleinman, "The Appeal of Experience; the Dismay of Images: Cultural Appropriations of Suffering in Our Times," *Daedalus* 125, no. 1 (1996): 1–23. James Agee puts forward his concern for this ethics of representation in his description of the Great Depression: "It seems to me curious, not to say obscene and thoroughly terrifying, that it could occur to an association of human beings drawn together through need and chance and for profit into a company, an organ of journalism, to pry intimately into the lives of an undefended and appallingly damaged group of human beings . . . in the name of science." James Agee and Walker Evans, *Let Us Now Praise Famous Men* (Boston: Houghton Mifflin, 1941), 5.

5 See Veena Das's response to Robbins that similarly rejects a distinction between a mode of anthropology attentive to suffering versus a mode of anthropology attuned to the good. Veena Das, *Affliction: Health, Disease, Poverty* (New York: Fordham University Press, 2015), 4.

6 On the imbrication of optimism and happiness as aiding rather than ameliorating suffering, see Sara Ahmed, *The Promise of Happiness* (Durham, NC: Duke University Press, 2010); Lauren Berlant, *Cruel Optimism* (Durham, NC: Duke University Press, 2011); Berlant, *Compassion: The Culture and Politics of an Emotion* (New York: Routledge, 2004). On the cognitive dissonance this produces in the context of the culture of cancer in the United States, see Lochlann Jain, *Malignant: How Cancer Becomes Us* (Berkeley: University of California Press, 2013).

7 Sandra Laugier, "Politics of Vulnerability and Responsibility for Ordinary Others," *Critical Horizons* 17, no. 2 (2016): 207–23.

8 For resonant conceptualizations of this form of violence, see Povinelli's "quasi-events," Nixon's "slow violence," and Berlant's "slow death." Elizabeth A. Po-

vinelli, *Economies of Abandonment: Social Belonging and Endurance in Late Liberalism* (Durham, NC: Duke University Press, 2011); Rob Nixon, *Slow Violence and the Environmentalism of the Poor* (Cambridge, MA: Harvard University Press, 2011); Lauren Berlant, "Slow Death (Sovereignty, Obesity, Lateral Agency)," *Critical Inquiry* 33, no. 4 (2007): 754–80.

9 In thinking of cancer as endemic, I draw upon Elizabeth Povinelli's understanding that "diseases of the poor" are not always "catastrophic or spectacular" but often also slow, chronic, and endemic. Povinelli, *Economies of Abandonment*, 134.

10 Ann Laura Stoler, *Duress: Imperial Durabilities in Our Times* (Durham, NC: Duke University Press, 2016).

11 In this sense, my understanding of endurance comes close to Jason Throop's conceptualization of "happiness" as a possible, precarious mode of being in a fragile world. But rather than presuppose the possibility of happiness, I take a more circumspect approach by taking up the conceptual language of endurance. C. Jason Throop, "Ambivalent Happiness and Virtuous Suffering," *HAU: Journal of Ethnographic Theory* 5, no. 3 (2015): 45–68.

12 R. Anuradha, "Deh ke Muhavre" [The idioms of the body], in *Adhoora Koi Nahin* (Delhi: Radhakrishna Prakashan, 2014), 18–19.

13 R. Anuradha, "Tum Na Badalna" [Don't you change], in *Adhoora Koi Nahin*, 20–21.

14 R. Anuradha, "Teri Meri Chup" [Our silence], in *Adhoora Koi Nahin*, 22.

15 Talal Asad, "Agency and Pain: An Exploration," *Culture and Religion* 1, no. 1 (2000): 29–60.

16 R. Anuradha, "Bhar do Mujhe" [Recognize me], in *Adhoora Koi Nahin*, 11.

17 R. Anuradha, "Rishte" [Relations], in *Adhoora Koi Nahin*, 61.

18 Clara Han, *Life in Debt: Times of Care and Violence in Neoliberal Chile* (Berkeley: University of California Press, 2012).

19 Wool, "In-Durable Sociality."

20 Adriana Petryna, *Life Exposed: Biological Citizens after Chernobyl* (Princeton, NJ: Princeton University Press, 2002); Nikolas Rose and Carlos Novas, "Biological Citizenship," in *Global Assemblages: Technology, Politics, Ethics as Anthropological Problems*, ed. Aiwha Ong and Stephen Collier (Malden, MA: Blackwell, 2005), 439–63.

21 Deborah Heath, Rayna Rapp, and Karen-Sue Taussig, "Genetic Citizenship," in *A Companion to the Anthropology of Politics*, ed. David Nugent and Joan Vincent (Malden, MA: Blackwell, 2008), 152–67.

22 Zoë H. Wool and Julie Livingston, "Collateral Afterworlds," *Social Text* 35, no. 1 (130) (2017): 1–15.

23 João Biehl and Peter Locke, "Foreword: Unfinished," in *Unfinished: The Anthropology of Becoming*, ed. João Biehl and Peter Locke (Durham, NC: Duke University Press, 2017), ix–xiii.

24 Biehl and Locke, "Foreword: Unfinished," x.

25 R. Anuradha, "Mutthi me ret" [A fistful of sand], in *Adhoora Koi Nahin*, 78.

BIBLIOGRAPHY

Agee, James, and Walker Evans. *Let Us Now Praise Famous Men*. Boston: Houghton Mifflin, 1941.

Agnes, Flavia. "The Supreme Court, the Media, and the Uniform Civil Code Debate in India." In *The Crisis of Secularism in India*, edited by Anuradha Dingwaney Needham and Rajeswari Sunder Rajan, 294–315. Durham, NC: Duke University Press, 2007.

Ahmed, Sara. *The Promise of Happiness*. Durham, NC: Duke University Press, 2010.

Alexander, P. John, Narayanakurup Dinesh, and M. S. Vidyasagar. "Psychiatric Morbidity among Cancer Patients and Its Relationship with Awareness of Illness and Expectations about Treatment Outcome." *Acta Oncologica* 32, no. 6 (1993): 623–26.

Amrith, Sunil. *Decolonizing International Health: India and Southeast Asia, 1930–65*. Basingstoke: Palgrave Macmillan, 2006.

Anand, B. K., G. S. Chinna, and B. Singh. "Studies on Shri Ramanand Yogi during His Stay in an Air-Tight Box." *Indian Journal of Medical Research* 49, no. 1 (1961): 82–89.

Anand, T., S. Grover, R. Kumar, M. Kumar, and G. K. Ingle. "Workplace Violence against Resident Doctors in a Tertiary Care Hospital in Delhi." *National Medical Journal of India* 29, no. 6 (2016): 344–48.

Anuradha, R. *Adhoora Koi Nahin*. Delhi: Radhakrishna Prakashan, 2014.

Asad, Talal. "Agency and Pain: An Exploration." *Culture and Religion* 1, no. 1 (2000): 29–60.

Badwe, R. A., R. Dikshit, M. Laversanne, and F. Bray. "Cancer Incidence Trends in India." *Japanese Journal of Clinical Oncology* 44, no. 5 (2014): 401–7.

Balhara, Yatan Pal Singh, Rajeev Ranjan, Anju Dhawan, and Deepak Yadav. "Experiences from a Community Based Substance Use Treatment Centre in an Urban Resettlement Colony in India." *Journal of Addiction* 2014 (2014): 1–6.

Banerjee, Dwaipayan. "Markets and Molecules: A Pharmaceutical Primer from the South." *Medical Anthropology* 36, no. 4 (2017): 363–80.

Baru, Rama V., A. Acharya, S. Acharya, Shiva Kumar, and K. Nagaraj. "Inequities in Access to Health Services in India: Caste, Class and Region." *Economic and Political Weekly* 45, no. 38 (2010): 49–58.

Basu, Srimati. "Judges of Normality: Mediating Marriage in the Family Courts of Kolkata, India." *Signs: Journal of Women in Culture and Society* 37, no. 2 (2012): 469–92.

Beegum, Nazeem. *My Mother Did Not Go Bald: Memoir of a Daughter.* Kottayam: Expressions, 2014.

Berlant, Lauren. *Compassion: The Culture and Politics of an Emotion.* New York: Routledge, 2004.

Berlant, Lauren. *Cruel Optimism.* Durham, NC: Duke University Press, 2011.

Berlant, Lauren. *The Female Complaint.* Durham, NC: Duke University Press, 2008.

Berlant, Lauren. "Slow Death (Sovereignty, Obesity, Lateral Agency)." *Critical Inquiry* 33, no. 4 (2007): 754–80.

Bhaskar, Ira. "Emotion, Subjectivity, and the Limits of Desire: Melodrama and Modernity in Bombay Cinema, 1940s–'50s." In *Gender Meets Genre in Postwar Cinemas,* edited by Christine Gledhill, 161–76. Urbana: University of Illinois Press, 2012.

Biehl, João. *Vita: Life in a Zone of Social Abandonment.* Berkeley: University of California Press, 2005.

Biehl, João, and Peter Locke. "Foreword: Unfinished." In *Unfinished: The Anthropology of Becoming,* edited by João Biehl and Peter Locke, ix–xiii. Durham, NC: Duke University Press, 2017.

Biehl, João, and Amy Moran-Thomas. "Symptom: Subjectivities, Social Ills, Technologies." *Annual Review of Anthropology* 38, no. 1 (2009): 267–88.

Boelstorff, Tom. "Nuri's Testimony: HIV/AIDS in Indonesia and Bare Knowledge." *American Ethnologist* 36, no. 2 (2009): 351–63.

Boltanski, Luc. *Distant Suffering: Morality, Media and Politics.* Cambridge: Cambridge University Press, 1999.

Broad, William J. *The Science of Yoga: The Risks and the Rewards.* New York: Simon and Schuster, 2012.

Brooks, Peter. *The Melodramatic Imagination: Balzac, Henry James, Melodrama, and the Mode of Excess.* New Haven, CT: Yale University Press, 1976.

Broom, Alex, and Assa Doron. "The Rise of Cancer in Urban India: Cultural Understandings, Structural Inequalities and the Emergence of the Clinic." *Health* 16, no. 3 (2012): 250–66.

Bruner, Jerome S. *Actual Minds, Possible Worlds.* Cambridge, MA: Harvard University Press, 1986.

Butler, Judith. *Antigone's Claim: Kinship between Life and Death.* New York: Columbia University Press, 2000.

Caduff, Carlo. *The Pandemic Perhaps: Dramatic Events in a Public Culture of Danger.* Berkeley: University of California Press, 2015.

"Cancer among Vegetarians." *British Medical Journal* 2, no. 1436 (1888): 29.

"Cancerous Trend." *Economic and Political Weekly* 32, no. 24 (1997): 1369.

Chakravarti, Uma. "From Fathers to Husbands: Of Love, Death and Marriage in North India." In *Honour Crimes, Paradigms, and Violence against Women,* edited by Lynn Welcgan and Sarah Hossain, 308–31. London: Zed Books, 2005.

Chandra, Prabha S., Santosh K. Chaturvedi, Anil Kumar, Sateesh Kumar, D. K. Subbakrishna, S. M. Channabasavanna, and N. Anantha. "Awareness of Diagnosis and Psychiatric Morbidity among Cancer Patients: A Study from South India." *Journal of Psychosomatic Research* 45, no. 3 (1998): 257–61.

Chandra, Prabha S., and Geetha Desai. "Denial as an Experiential Phenomenon in Serious Illness." *Indian Journal of Palliative Care* 13, no. 1 (2007): 8–14.

Chatterji, Shoma. "Hrishikesh Mukherjee: Giving Cinema a New Definition." *Silhouette*, September 30, 2015. https://learningandcreativity.com/silhouette/hrishikesh-mukherjee-interview/.

Chaturvedi, Santosh K. "Ethical Dilemmas in Palliative Care in Traditional Developing Societies, with Special Reference to the Indian Setting." *Journal of Medical Ethics* 34, no. 8 (2008): 611–15.

Chaturvedi, Santosh K. "Spiritual Issues at End of Life." *Indian Journal of Palliative Care* 13, no. 2 (2007): 48–52.

Chaturvedi, Santosh K. "What's Important for Quality of Life to Indians—in Relation to Cancer." *Social Science and Medicine* 33, no. 1 (1991): 91–94.

Chaturvedi, Santosh K., Carmen G. Loiselle, and Prabha S. Chandra. "Communication with Relatives and Collusion in Palliative Care: A Cross-Cultural Perspective." *Indian Journal of Palliative Care* 15, no. 1 (2009): 2–9.

Chaudhry, Minakshi. *Sunshine: My Encounter with Cancer*. New Delhi: Rupa, 2011.

Chittem, Mahati, Paul Norman, and Peter R. Harris. "Relationships between Perceived Diagnostic Disclosure, Patient Characteristics, Psychological Distress and Illness Perceptions in Indian Cancer Patients." *Psycho-Oncology* 22, no. 6 (2013): 1375–80.

Chua, Jocelyn Lim. "The Register of 'Complaint': Psychiatric Diagnosis and the Discourse of Grievance in the South Indian Mental Health Encounter." *Medical Anthropology Quarterly* 26, no. 2 (2012): 221–40.

Cohen, Lawrence. "Foreign Operations: Reflections on Clinical Mobility in Indian Film and Beyond." In *Critical Mobilities*, edited by Ola Soderstrom, Didier Ruedin, Shalini Randeria, Gianni D'Amato, and Francesco Panese, 213–34. Abingdon, UK: Routledge, 2013.

Cohen, Lawrence. *No Aging in India: Alzheimer's, the Bad Family, and Other Modern Things*. Berkeley: University of California Press, 1998.

Comaroff, Jean, and John L. Comaroff. *Theory from the South: Or, How Euro-America Is Evolving toward Africa*. London: Paradigm, 2012.

Conway, Kathlyn. *Beyond Words: Illness and the Limits of Expression*. Albuquerque: University of New Mexico Press, 2013.

Conway, Kathlyn. *Ordinary Life: A Memoir of Illness*. Ann Arbor: University of Michigan Press, 2007.

Copeman, Jacob, and Dwaipayan Banerjee. *Hematologies: The Political Life of Blood in India*. Ithaca, NY: Cornell University Press, 2019.

Crawford, S. Cromwell. *Dilemmas of Life and Death: Hindu Ethics in North American Context*. Albany, NY: SUNY Press, 1995.

Crawford, S. Cromwell. *The Evolution of Hindu Ethical Ideals*. Manoa: University of Hawaii Press, 1974.

Crawford, S. Cromwell. *Hindu Bioethics for the Twenty-First Century*. Albany, NY: SUNY Press, 2003.

Dalal, Ajit K. "Living with a Chronic Disease: Healing and Psychological Adjustment in Indian Society." *Psychology and Developing Societies* 12, no. 1 (2000): 67–81.

Darne, Padmakar. "Misconceptions about Cancer Therapy." *Economic and Political Weekly* 12, no. 44 (1977): 1844–45.

Das, Veena. *Affliction: Health, Disease, Poverty.* New York: Fordham University Press, 2015.

Das, Veena. "The Dreamed Guru: The Entangled Lives of the Amil and the Anthropologist." In *The Guru in South Asia*, edited by Jacob Copeman and Aya Ikegame, 144–66. Abingdon, UK: Routledge, 2012.

Das, Veena. *Life and Words: Violence and the Descent into the Ordinary.* Berkeley: University of California Press, 2007.

Das, Veena. "Ordinary Ethics." In *A Companion to Moral Anthropology*, edited by Didier Fassin, 133–49. Malden, MA: Wiley-Blackwell, 2012.

Das, Veena. "Violence and Nonviolence at the Heart of Hindu Ethics." In *The Oxford Handbook of Religion and Violence*, edited by Michael Jerryson, Mark Juergensmeyer, and Margo Kitts, 15–40. Oxford: Oxford University Press, 2013.

Das, Veena. "War and the Mythological Imagination." *Antropologia*, no. 16 (2013): 25–35.

Das, Veena. "What Does Ordinary Ethics Look Like?" In *Four Lectures on Ethics*, edited by Michael Lambek, Veena Das, Didier Fassin, and Webb Keane, 53–127. Chicago: HAU Books, 2015.

Das, Veena, and Ranendra Kumar Das. *The Interface between Mental Health and Reproductive Health of Women among the Urban Poor in Delhi.* Thiruvananthapuram: Achutha Menon Centre for Health Science Studies, Sree Chitra Tirunal Institute for Medical Sciences and Technology, 2005.

Davis, Mark, and Lenore Manderson. *Disclosure in Health and Illness.* London: Routledge, 2014.

Dayal, Prabhoo, and Yatan Pal Singh Balhara. "Profile of Female Patients Seeking In-Patient Treatment for Prescription Opioid Abuse from a Tertiary Care Drug Dependence Treatment Centre from India." *Indian Journal of Medical Research* 143, no. 1 (2016): 95–100.

Deshpande, Sudhavna. "The Consumable Hero of Globalized India." In *Bollyworld: Popular Indian Cinema through a Transnational Lens*, edited by Raminder Kaur and Ajay Sinha, 186–203. New Delhi: Sage, 2005.

Dhillon, Preet K., Prashant Mathur, A. Nandakumar, Christina Fitzmaurice, G. Anil Kumar, Ravi Mehrotra, D. K. Shukla, et al. "The Burden of Cancers and Their Variations across the States of India: The Global Burden of Disease Study 1990–2016." *Lancet Oncology* 19, no. 10 (2018): 1289–306.

Dirks, Nicholas B. *Castes of Mind: Colonialism and the Making of Modern India.* Princeton, NJ: Princeton University Press, 2001.

Doane, Mary Ann. *The Desire to Desire: The Woman's Film of the 1940s.* Bloomington: Indiana University Press, 1987.

Doniger, Wendy. *On Hinduism.* Oxford: Oxford University Press, 2014.

Ecks, Stefan. "Global Pharmaceutical Markets and Corporate Citizenship: The Case of Novartis' Anti-cancer Drug Glivec." *BioSocieties* 3 (2008): 165–81.

Eysenck, H. J. "Cancer, Personality and Stress: Prediction and Prevention." *Advances in Behaviour Research and Therapy* 16, no. 3 (1994): 167–215.

Farmer, P., J. Frenk, F. M. Knaul, L. N. Shulman, G. Alleyne, L. Armstrong, R. Atun, et al. "Expansion of Cancer Care and Control in Countries of Low and Middle Income: A Call to Action." *Lancet* 376, no. 9747 (2010): 1186–93.

Finkel, Madelon Lubin. *Cancer Screening in the Developing World: Case Studies and Strategies from the Field.* Hanover, NH: Dartmouth College Press, 2018.

Firth, S. "End-of-Life: A Hindu View." *Lancet* 366, no. 9486 (2005): 682–86.

Fischer, Michael M. J. "Urban Mahabharata: Health Care, Ordinary, Traditional, and Contemporary Ethics." *Medicine Anthropology Theory* 4, no. 3 (2017): 98–129.

Foucault, Michel. "17 March 1976." In *"Society Must Be Defended": Lectures at the Collège De France, 1975–1976,* edited by David Macey, 239–64. New York: Picador, 2003.

François, Anne-Lise. *Open Secrets: The Literature of Uncounted Experience.* Stanford, CA: Stanford University Press, 2008.

Frank, Arthur W. *The Wounded Storyteller: Body, Illness, and Ethics.* Chicago: University of Chicago Press, 1995.

Ganti, Tejaswini. *Producing Bollywood: Inside the Contemporary Hindi Film Industry.* Durham, NC: Duke University Press, 2012.

Ganti, Tejaswini. "Sentiments of Disdain and Practices of Distinction: Boundary-Work, Subjectivity, and Value in the Hindi Film Industry." *Anthropological Quarterly* 85, no. 1 (2012): 5–43.

Gawande, Atul. *Being Mortal: Medicine and What Matters in the End.* New York: Metropolitan Books, 2014.

George, Mathew Sunil, and Helen Lambert. "'I Am Doing Fine Only Because I Have Not Told Anyone': The Necessity of Concealment in the Lives of People Living with HIV in India." *Culture, Health and Sexuality* 17, no. 8 (2015): 933–46.

Gledhill, Christine. "The Melodramatic Field: An Investigation." In *Home Is Where the Heart Is: Studies in Melodrama and the Woman's Film,* edited by Christine Gledhill, 5–39. London: BFI Publishing, 1987.

Goffman, Erving. *Stigma: Notes on the Management of Spoiled Identity.* New York: J. Aronson, 1974.

Good, Byron J., Mary-Jo DelVecchio Good, Isenbike Togan, Zafer Ilbars, A. Güvener, and Ilker Gelişen. "In the Subjunctive Mode: Epilepsy Narratives in Turkey." *Social Science and Medicine* 38, no. 6 (1994): 835–42.

Good, Mary-Jo DelVecchio, Byron J. Good, Cynthia Schaffer, and Stuart E. Lind. "American Oncology and the Discourse on Hope." *Culture, Medicine and Psychiatry* 14, no. 1 (1990): 59–79.

Good, Mary-Jo DelVecchio, Sandra Theresa Hyde, Sarah Pinto, and Byron J. Good. *Postcolonial Disorders.* Berkeley: University of California Press, 2008.

Gooptu, Nandini. "New Spirituality, Politics of Self-Empowerment, Citizenship, and Democracy in Contemporary India." *Modern Asian Studies* 50, no. 3 (2016): 934–74.

Goudas, Leonidas C., Rina Bloch, Maria Gialeli-Goudas, Joseph Lau, and Daniel B. Carr. "The Epidemiology of Cancer Pain." *Cancer Investigation* 23, no. 2 (2005): 182–90.

Graham, Fiona, and David Clark. "Definition and Evaluation: Developing the Debate on Community Participation in Palliative Care." *Indian Journal of Palliative Care* 11, no. 1 (2005): 2–5.

Grover, Shalini. *Marriage, Love, Caste, and Kinship Support: Lived Experiences of the Urban Poor in India.* New Delhi: Social Science Press, 2011.

Gulia, S., M. Sengar, R. Badwe, and S. Gupta. "National Cancer Control Programme in India: Proposal for Organization of Chemotherapy and Systemic Therapy Services." *Journal of Global Oncology* 3, no. 3 (2017): 271–74.

Gupta, Harmala. "Community Participation in Palliative Care: A Comment." *Indian Journal of Palliative Care* 11, no. 1 (2005): 19–21.

Gupta, Harmala. "A Journey from Cancer to 'Cansupport.'" *Indian Journal of Palliative Care* 10, no. 1 (2004): 32–38.

Hacking, Ian. "Making Up People." In *Reconstructing Individualism: Autonomy, Individuality and Self in Western Thought,* edited by Thomas C. Heller, Morton Sosna, and David Wellbery, 222–36. Stanford, CA: Stanford University Press, 1986.

Haider, Saraswati. "Migrant Women and Urban Experience in a Squatter Settlement." In *Delhi: Urban Space and Human Destinies,* edited by Veronique Dupont, Emma Tarlo, and Denis Vidal, 29–49. New Delhi: Manohar, 2000.

Hammer, Sheila L., Karen Clark, Marcia Grant, and Matthew J. Loscalzo. "Seventeen Years of Progress for Supportive Care Services: A Resurvey of National Cancer Institute–Designated Comprehensive Cancer Centers." *Palliative and Supportive Care* 13, no. 4 (2015): 917–25.

Han, Clara. *Life in Debt: Times of Care and Violence in Neoliberal Chile.* Berkeley: University of California Press, 2012.

Han, Clara. "Symptoms of Another Life: Time, Possibility, and Domestic Relations in Chile's Credit Economy." *Cultural Anthropology* 26, no. 1 (2011): 7–32.

Hansen, Helena, and Mary E. Skinner. "From White Bullets to Black Markets and Greened Medicine: The Neuroeconomics and Neuroracial Politics of Opioid Pharmaceuticals." *Annals of Anthropological Practice* 36, no. 1 (2012): 167–82.

Hawkins, Anne. "Pathography: Patient Narratives of Illness." *Western Journal of Medicine* 171, no. 2 (1999): 127–29.

Heath, Deborah, Rayna Rapp, and Karen-Sue Taussig. "Genetic Citizenship." In *A Companion to the Anthropology of Politics,* edited by David Nugent and Joan Vincent, 152–67. Malden, MA: Blackwell, 2008.

Hinze, Susan W. "Gender and the Body of Medicine or at Least Some Body Parts: (Re)Constructing the Prestige Hierarchy of Medical Specialties." *Sociological Quarterly* 40, no. 2 (1999): 217–39.

Hoffman, Frederick I. "Cancer in India, Persia and Ceylon." *Sankhyā: The Indian Journal of Statistics (1933–1960)* 2, no. 3 (1936): 281–306.

Holmes, David. "A Disease of Growth." *Nature* 521, no. 7551 (2015): s2–s3.

Holmes, Douglas R., and George E. Marcus. "Para-Ethnography." In *The Sage Encyclopedia of Qualitative Research Methods,* edited by Lisa Given, 595–97. Thousand Oaks, CA: Sage, 2008.

Hui, D., A. Elsayem, M. De la Cruz, A. Berger, D. S. Zhukovsky, S. Palla, A. Evans, N.

Fadul, J. L. Palmer, and E. Bruera. "Availability and Integration of Palliative Care at US Cancer Centers." *JAMA* 303, no. 11 (2010): 1054–61.

IANS. "Sanjay Dutt Gets Teary Eyed; Recalls Nargis Dutt's Fight against Cancer." *DNA* India. Accessed December 7, 2019. http://www.dnaindia.com/entertainment/report-sanjay-dutt-gets-teary-eyed-recalls-nargis-dutt-s-fight-against-cancer-1771416.

International Agency for Research on Cancer. "Globocan 2018: All Cancers Fact Sheet." Accessed December 7, 2019. http://gco.iarc.fr/today/data/factsheets/cancers/39-All-cancers-fact-sheet.pdf.

Isaac, Thomas, and Richard Franke. *Local Democracy and Development: The Kerala People's Campaign for Decentralized Planning.* Lanham, MD: Rowman and Littlefield, 2002.

Jackson, Jean E. *"Camp Pain": Talking with Chronic Cancer Patients.* Philadelphia: University of Pennsylvania Press, 2000.

Jain, Lochlann. *Malignant: How Cancer Becomes Us.* Berkeley: University of California Press, 2013.

Jana, Smarajit. "Community Mobilisation: Myths and Challenges." *Journal of Epidemiology and Community Health* 66, no. 2 (2012): ii5–ii6.

Jesudasan, Usha. *Two Journeys: The Challenges of Breast Cancer.* Bengaluru: Berean Bay Media House, 2016.

Jeter, Pamela, Jerry Slutsky, Nilkamal Singh, and Sat Bir Khalsa. "Yoga as a Therapeutic Intervention: A Bibliometric Analysis of Published Research Studies from 1967 to 2013." *Journal of Alternative and Complementary Medicine* 21, no. 10 (2015): 586–92.

Jones, David, and Jeremy Greene. "The Decline and Rise of Coronary Heart Disease: Understanding Public Health Catastrophism." *American Journal of Public Health* 103, no. 7 (2013): 1207–18.

Jurecic, Ann. *Illness as Narrative.* Pittsburgh: University of Pittsburgh Press, 2012.

Kalanithi, Paul. *When Breath Becomes Air.* New York: Random House, 2016.

Kandasamy, A., S. K. Chaturvedi, and G. Desai. "Spirituality, Distress, Depression, Anxiety, and Quality of Life in Patients with Advanced Cancer." *Indian Journal of Cancer* 48, no. 1 (2011): 55–59.

Kastor, Anshul, and Sanjay K. Mohanty. "Disease-Specific Out-of-Pocket and Catastrophic Health Expenditure on Hospitalization in India: Do Indian Households Face Distress Health Financing?" *PLoS One* 13, no. 5 (2018): e0196106.

Kelly, Tobias. "A Life Less Miserable?" *HAU: Journal of Ethnographic Theory* 3, no. 1 (2013): 213–16.

Kleinman, Arthur, and Joan Kleinman. "The Appeal of Experience; the Dismay of Images: Cultural Appropriations of Suffering in Our Times." *Daedalus* 125, no. 1 (1996): 1–23.

Knauft, Bruce. "Good Anthropology in Dark Times: Critical Appraisal and Ethnographic Application." *Australian Journal of Anthropology* 30 (2018): 3–17.

Knaul, Felicia Marie, Paul E. Farmer, Eric L. Krakauer, Liliana De Lima, Afsan Bhadelia, Xiaoxiao Jiang Kwete, Héctor Arreola-Ornelas, et al. "Alleviating the

Access Abyss in Palliative Care and Pain Relief—an Imperative of Universal Health Coverage: The Lancet Commission Report." *Lancet* 391, no. 10128 (2018): 1391–454.

Kohli, Neena, and Ajit K. Dalal. "Culture as a Factor in Causal Understanding of Illness: A Study of Cancer Patients." *Psychology and Developing Societies* 10, no. 2 (1998): 115–29.

Koshy, Cherian. "The Palliative Care Movement in India: Another Freedom Struggle or a Silent Revolution?" *Indian Journal of Palliative Care* 15, no. 1 (2009): 10–13.

Kowalski, Julia. "Ordering Dependence: Care, Disorder, and Kinship Ideology in North Indian Antiviolence Counseling." *American Ethnologist* 43, no. 1 (2016): 63–75.

Kulick, Don. "Theory in Furs: Masochist Anthropology." *Current Anthropology* 47, no. 6 (2006): 933–52.

Kumar, Anup. *The Joy of Cancer*. New Delhi: Rupa, 2002.

Kumar, Neelam. *To Cancer, with Love: My Journey of Joy*. Delhi: Hay House, 2015.

Kumar, Suresh, and Mathews Numpeli. "Neighborhood Network in Palliative Care." *Indian Journal of Palliative Care* 11, no. 1 (2005): 6–9.

Laidlaw, James. "For an Anthropology of Ethics and Freedom." *Journal of the Royal Anthropological Institute* 8, no. 2 (2002): 311–32.

Lamb, Sarah. *White Saris and Sweet Mangoes: Aging, Gender, and Body in North India*. Berkeley: University of California Press, 2000.

Laugier, Sandra. "Politics of Vulnerability and Responsibility for Ordinary Others." *Critical Horizons* 17, no. 2 (2016): 207–23.

Lemons, Katherine. "The Politics of Livability: Tutoring 'Kinwork' in a New Delhi Women's Arbitration Center." *PoLAR: Political and Legal Anthropology Review* 39, no. 2 (2016): 244–60.

Lind, Stuart E., Mary-Jo DelVecchio Good, Steven Seidel, Thomas Csordas, and Byron J. Good. "Telling the Diagnosis of Cancer." *Journal of Clinical Oncology* 7, no. 5 (1989): 583–89.

Livingston, Julie. *Improvising Medicine: An African Oncology Ward in an Emerging Cancer Epidemic*. Durham, NC: Duke University Press, 2012.

Lukhmana, S., S. Bhasin, P. Chhabra, and M. Bhatia. "Family Caregivers' Burden: A Hospital Based Study in 2010 among Cancer Patients from Delhi." *Indian Journal of Cancer* 52, no. 1 (2015): 146–51.

Luzzati, T., A. Parenti, and T. Rughi. "Economic Growth and Cancer Incidence." *Ecological Economics* 146 (2018): 381–96.

Lynch, Thomas, Stephen Connor, and David Clark. "Mapping Levels of Palliative Care Development: A Global Update." *Journal of Pain and Symptom Management* 45, no. 6 (2013): 1094–106.

Madan, T. N. "Community Involvement in Health Policy: Socio-structural and Dynamic Aspects of Health Beliefs." *Social Science and Medicine* 25, no. 6 (1987): 615–20.

Magrath, Ian. "Cancer in Low- and Middle-Income Countries." In *Health G20*, edited by Manuel Carballo, 58–68. Sutton, UK: Pro-Brook, 2010.

Maheshwari, Anand Prakash. *Mayan*. Delhi: Prabhat Prakashan, 2012.

Malhotra, Amita. *Silent Echoes: A True Story*. New Delhi: New Dawn, 2005.

"Malignant Disease in India." *British Medical Journal* 1, no. 3926 (1936): 718–19.

Mallath, Mohandas K., David G. Taylor, Rajendra A. Badwe, Goura K. Rath, V. Shanta, C. S. Pramesh, Raghunadharao Digumarti, et al. "The Growing Burden of Cancer in India: Epidemiology and Social Context." *Lancet Oncology* 15, no. 6 (2014): e205–e212.

Mani, Lata. "Production of an Official Discourse on 'Sati' in Early Nineteenth Century Bengal." *Economic and Political Weekly* 21, no. 17 (1986): 32–40.

Martin, Emily. *Bipolar Expeditions: Mania and Depression in American Culture*. Princeton, NJ: Princeton University Press, 2007.

Martis, Lawrence, and Anne Westhues. "A Synthesis of the Literature on Breaking Bad News or Truth Telling: Potential for Research in India." *Indian Journal of Palliative Care* 19, no. 1 (2013): 2–11.

McDermott, Elizabeth, Lucy Selman, Michael Wright, and David Clark. "Hospice and Palliative Care Development in India: A Multimethod Review of Services and Experiences." *Journal of Pain and Symptom Management* 35, no. 6 (2008): 583–93.

McDowell, Andrew. "Mohit's Pharmakon: Symptom, Rotational Bodies, and Pharmaceuticals in Rural Rajasthan." *Medical Anthropology Quarterly* 31, no. 3 (2017): 332–48.

McMullin, Juliet. "Cancer." *Annual Review of Anthropology* 45, no. 1 (2016): 251–66.

McMullin, Juliet. "Cancer and the Comics: Graphic Narratives and Biolegitimate Lives." *Medical Anthropology Quarterly* 30, no. 2 (2016): 149–67.

Melzack, Ronald, and Patrick Wall. "Pain Mechanisms: A New Theory." *Science* 150, no. 3699 (1965): 971–79.

Metcalf, Peter, and Richard Huntington. *Celebrations of Death: The Anthropology of Mortuary Ritual*. Cambridge: Cambridge University Press, 1991.

Mill, James. *The History of British India*. London: Printed for Baldwin, Cradock, and Joy, 1817.

Moran-Thomas, Amy. "Metabola: Chronic Disease and Damaged Life in Belize." PhD diss., Princeton University, 2012.

Moran-Thomas, Amy. "Struggles for Maintenance: Patient Activism and Dialysis Dilemmas amidst a Global Diabetes Epidemic." *Global Public Health* 14, nos. 6–7 (2019): 1044–57.

Morgan, Lynn M. "Community Participation in Health: Perpetual Allure, Persistent Challenge." *Health Policy and Planning* 16, no. 3 (2001): 221–30.

Mrs 55. "Lymphosarcoma of the Intestine: The Making of a Bollywood Legend." *Mr. and Mrs. 55—Classic Bollywood Revisited*, February 20, 2012. https://mrandmrs55.com/2012/02/20/lymphosarcoma-of-the-intestine-the-making-of-a-bollywood-legend/.

Mueller, Lucas M. "Cancer in the Tropics: Geographical Pathology and the Formation of Cancer Epidemiology." *BioSocieties* 14, no. 4 (2019): 512–28.

Mukharji, Projit Bihari. *Doctoring Traditions: Ayurveda, Small Technologies, and Braided Sciences*. Chicago: University of Chicago Press, 2016.

Muller, F. Max. *India, What Can It Teach Us? A Course of Lectures.* London: Longmans, Green, 1883.

Nath, Vishwa, and Khem Singh Grewal. "Cancer in India." *Indian Journal of Medical Research* 23, no. 1 (1935): 149–90.

Nixon, Rob. *Slow Violence and the Environmentalism of the Poor.* Cambridge, MA: Harvard University Press, 2011.

Nyblade, L., M. Stockton, S. Travasso, and S. Krishnan. "A Qualitative Exploration of Cervical and Breast Cancer Stigma in Karnataka, India." *BMC Women's Health* 17, no. 1 (2017): 1–15.

Omran, Abdul. "The Epidemiologic Transition: A Theory of the Epidemiology of Population Change." *Milbank Memorial Fund Quarterly* 49, no. 4 (1971): 509–38.

Ortner, Sherry B. "Dark Anthropology and Its Others." *HAU: Journal of Ethnographic Theory* 6, no. 1 (2016): 47–73.

Palriwala, Rajni, and Ravinder Kaur. "Marriage in South Asia: Continuities and Transformations." In *Marrying in South Asia: Shifting Concepts, Changing Practices in a Globalizing World*, edited by Rajni Palriwala and Ravinder Kaur, 1–27. Delhi: Orient Blackswan, 2014.

Pandve, Harshal. "Cancer and Indian Films." *Journal of Cancer Research and Therapeutics* 6, no. 2 (2010): 233.

Pati, Sanghamitra. "Bollywood's Cancer: Disconnect between Reel and Real Oncology." *Cancer and Society* 16, no. 8 (2015): 894–95.

Petryna, Adriana. *Life Exposed: Biological Citizens after Chernobyl.* Princeton, NJ: Princeton University Press, 2002.

Pinto, Sarah. *Daughters of Parvati: Women and Madness in Contemporary India.* Philadelphia: University of Pennsylvania Press, 2014.

Pinto, Sarah. *The Doctor and Mrs. A.: Ethics and Counter-ethics in an Indian Dream Analysis.* New York: Fordham University Press, 2019.

Pinto, Sarah. *Where There Is No Midwife: Birth and Loss in Rural India.* New York: Berghahn Books, 2008.

Pocock, D. F. "Preservation of the Religious Life: Hindu Immigrants in England." *Contributions to Indian Sociology* 10, no. 2 (1976): 341–65.

Polanyi, Michael. *The Tacit Dimension.* London: Routledge, 1967.

Povinelli, Elizabeth A. *Economies of Abandonment: Social Belonging and Endurance in Late Liberalism.* Durham, NC: Duke University Press, 2011.

Povinelli, Elizabeth A. *The Empire of Love: Toward a Theory of Intimacy, Genealogy, and Carnality.* Durham, NC: Duke University Press, 2006.

Prasad, Madhava. "Diverting Diseases." In *Figurations in Indian Film*, edited by Anustup Basu and Meheli Sen, 91–100. London: Palgrave Macmillan, 2013.

Price, Reynolds. *A Whole New Life: An Illness and a Healing.* New York: Scribner, 2003.

Purakkal, D., D. Pulassery, and S. Ravindran. "Should a Patient with a Life Threatening Illness Be Informed of the Diagnosis? A Survey of Physicians and Medical Students in Calicut." *Indian Journal of Palliative Care* 10, no. 2 (2004): 64–66.

Rajagopal, M. R., and David E. Joranson. "India: Opioid Availability; an Update." *Journal of Pain and Symptom Management* 33, no. 5 (2007): 615–22.

Rajan, Kaushik Sunder. "The Experimental Machinery of Global Clinical Trials: Case Studies from India." *Asian Biotech* 38, no. 1 (2010): 55–80.

Rajpal, Sunil, Abhishek Kumar, and William Joe. "Economic Burden of Cancer in India: Evidence from Cross-Sectional Nationally Representative Household Survey, 2014." *PloS One* 13, no. 2 (2018): 1–17.

Rapp, Rayna. "The Thick Social Matrix for Bioethics: Anthropological Approaches." In *Bioethics in Cultural Contexts*, edited by Marcus Well, Dietmar Mieth, and Christoph Rehmann-Sutter, 341–51. Dordrecht: Springer Netherlands, 2006.

"Recurrence of Malignant Growths after Removal." *British Medical Journal* 1, no. 1423 (1888): 761.

Reddy, Vijay Anand. *I Am a Survivor*. New Delhi: Penguin Random House India, 2017.

Rifkin, Susan B. "Paradigms Lost: Toward a New Understanding of Community Participation in Health Programmes." *Acta Tropica* 61, no. 2 (1996): 79–92.

Robbins, Joel. "Beyond the Suffering Subject: Toward an Anthropology of the Good." *Journal of the Royal Anthropological Institute* 19, no. 3 (2013): 447–62.

Rose, Nikolas, and Carlos Novas. "Biological Citizenship." In *Global Assemblages: Technology, Politics, Ethics as Anthropological Problems*, edited by Aiwha Ong and Stephen Collier, 439–63. Malden, MA: Blackwell, 2005.

Roth, Ram, Elizabeth A. M. Frost, Clifford Gevirtz, and Carrie L. H. Atcheson. *The Role of Anesthesiology in Global Health: A Comprehensive Guide*. New York: Springer, 2015.

Roy, Srirupa. *Beyond Belief: India and the Politics of Postcolonial Nationalism*. Durham, NC: Duke University Press, 2007.

Ruddock, Anna Louise. "Special Medicine: Producing Doctors at the All India Institute of Medical Sciences (AIIMS)." PhD diss., King's College London, 2017.

Saha, Moitreyee. *My Date with Cancer*. Gurgaon: Partridge, 2014.

Sangari, Kumkum. "Violent Acts: Cultures, Structures and Retraditionalisation." In *Women of India: Colonial and Post-colonial Periods*, edited by Bharati Ray, 159–81. Delhi: Sage, 2005.

Saria, Vaibhav. "To Be Some Other Name: The Naming Games That Hijras Play." *South Asia Multidisciplinary Academic Journal*, no. 12 (2015): 1–16.

Sarin, Rajiv. "Indian National Cancer Control Programme: Setting Sight on Shifting Targets." *Journal of Cancer Research and Therapeutics* 1, no. 4 (2005): 240–48.

Scarry, Elaine. *The Body in Pain: The Making and Unmaking of the World*. New York: Oxford University Press, 1985.

Scheffler, Robin Wolfe. *A Contagious Cause: The American Hunt for Cancer Viruses and the Rise of Molecular Medicine*. Chicago: University of Chicago Press, 2019.

Seligman, Adam, Robert Weller, Michael Puett, and Bennett Simon. *Ritual and Its Consequences: An Essay on the Limits of Sincerity*. Oxford: Oxford University Press, 2008.

Simmel, Georg. "The Sociology of Secrecy and of Secret Societies." *American Journal of Sociology* 11, no. 4 (1906): 441–98.

Singer, M. B. *When a Great Tradition Modernizes*. Chicago: University of Chicago Press, 1972.

Singh, Amita Tyagi, and Patricia Uberoi. "Learning to 'Adjust': Conjugal Relations in Indian Popular Fiction." *Bulletin (Centre for Women's Development Studies)* 1, no. 1 (1994): 93–120.

Singh, Holly Donahue. "Fertility Control: Reproductive Desires, Kin Work, and Women's Status in Contemporary India." *Medical Anthropology Quarterly* 31, no. 1 (2017): 23–39.

Sivaramakrishnan, Kavita. *As the World Ages: Rethinking a Demographic Crisis.* Cambridge, MA: Harvard University Press, 2018.

Sivaramakrishnan, Kavita. "Global Histories of Health, Disease, and Medicine from a 'Zig-Zag' Perspective." *Bulletin of the History of Medicine* 89, no. 4 (2015): 700–704.

Snell-Rood, Claire Natalie. *No One Will Let Her Live: Women's Struggle for Well-Being in a Delhi Slum.* Oakland: University of California Press, 2015.

Solomon, Harris. *Metabolic Living: Food, Fat, and the Absorption of Illness in India.* Durham, NC: Duke University Press, 2016.

Sontag, Susan. AIDS *and Its Metaphors.* New York: Farrar, Straus and Giroux, 1989.

Sontag, Susan. *Illness as Metaphor.* New York: Farrar, Straus and Giroux, 1978.

Srinath Reddy, K., Bela Shah, Cherian Varghese, and Anbumani Ramadoss. "Responding to the Threat of Chronic Diseases in India." *Lancet* 366, no. 9498 (2005): 1744–49.

Srinivas, Tulasi. "Artful Living." In *Critical Themes in Indian Sociology*, edited by Sanjay Srivastava, Yasmeen Arif, and Janaki Abraham, 62–76. New Delhi: Sage, 2018.

Stevenson, Lisa. *Life beside Itself: Imagining Care in the Canadian Arctic.* Oakland: University of California Press, 2014.

Stjernswärd, Jan. "Community Participation in Palliative Care." *Indian Journal of Palliative Care* 11, no. 1 (2005): 22–27.

Stoler, Ann Laura. *Duress: Imperial Durabilities in Our Times.* Durham, NC: Duke University Press, 2016.

Stoler, Ann Laura. "Imperial Debris: Reflections on Ruins and Ruination." *Cultural Anthropology* 23, no. 2 (2008): 191–219.

Subramanian, Ajantha. "Making Merit: The Indian Institutes of Technology and the Social Life of Caste." *Comparative Studies in Society and History* 57, no. 2 (2015): 291–322.

Thomas, B., Manoj Pandey, K. Ramdas, and Muthu Nair. "Psychological Distress in Cancer Patients: Hypothesis of a Distress Model." *European Journal of Cancer Prevention* 11, no. 2 (2002): 179–85.

Thresia, C. U. "Rising Private Sector and Falling 'Good Health at Low Cost': Health Challenges in China, Sri Lanka, and Indian State of Kerala." *International Journal of Health Services* 43, no. 1 (2013): 31–48.

Throop, C. Jason. "Ambivalent Happiness and Virtuous Suffering." HAU: *Journal of Ethnographic Theory* 5, no. 3 (2015): 45–68.

Ticktin, Miriam. "Transnational Humanitarianism." *Review of Anthropology* 43, no. 1 (2014): 273–89.

Torre, Lindsey A., Rebecca L. Siegel, Elizabeth M. Ward, and Ahmedin Jemal. "Global Cancer Incidence and Mortality Rates and Trends: An Update." *Cancer Epidemiology, Biomarkers and Prevention* 25, no. 1 (2016): 16–27.

Tripathi, Kamlesh. *Gloom behind the Smile.* New Delhi: Pigeon Books, 2012.

Unkule, Nitin. *Cancer Care and Mysteries and Yoga.* Pune, Maharashtra: Mehta, 2010.

van den Beuken–van Everdingen, Marieke H. J., Laura M. J. Hochstenbach, Elbert A. J. Joosten, Vivianne C. G. Tjan-Heijnen, and Daisy J. A. Janssen. "Update on Prevalence of Pain in Patients with Cancer: Systematic Review and Meta-analysis." *Journal of Pain and Symptom Management* 51, no. 6 (2016): 1070–90.

Van Hollen, Cecilia. *Birth on the Threshold: Childbirth and Modernity in South India.* Berkeley: University of California Press, 2003.

Van Hollen, Cecilia. "Handle with Care: Rethinking the Rights versus Culture Dichotomy in Cancer Disclosure in India." *Medical Anthropology Quarterly* 32, no. 1 (2018): 59–84.

Van Hollen, Cecilia. "Nationalism, Transnationalism, and the Politics of 'Traditional' Indian Medicine for HIV/AIDS." In *Asian Medicine and Globalization,* edited by Joseph S. Alter, 88–106. Philadelphia: University of Pennsylvania Press, 2005.

Varghese, Cherian. "Cancer Prevention and Control in India." In *50 Years of Cancer Control in India,* edited by Indian Department of Health, 48–59. New Delhi: Indian Department of Health, 2003.

Varghese, Mammen. *Upgraded to Life.* Bangalore: Pothi, 2016.

Varma, Saiba. "The Medical Net: Patients, Psychiatrists and Paper Trails in the Kashmir Valley." PhD diss., Cornell University, 2013.

Vasudevan, Ravi. *The Melodramatic Public: Film Form and Spectatorship in Indian Cinema.* Ranikhet: Permanent Black, 2011.

Vasudevan, S. "Coping with Terminal Illness: A Spiritual Perspective." *Indian Journal of Palliative Care* 9, no. 1 (2003): 19–24.

Vatuk, Sylvia. "The 'Women's Court' in India: An Alternative Dispute Resolution Body for Women in Distress." *Journal of Legal Pluralism and Unofficial Law* 45, no. 1 (2013): 76–103.

Venkat, Bharat. "Cures." *Public Culture* 28, no. 3 (80) (2016): 475–97.

Venkatesh, Roopa. *Cancer: A Comma, Not a Fullstop.* New Delhi: Shroff, 2013.

Waghorne, Joanne Punzo. "Engineering an Artful Practice: On Jaggi Vasudev's Isha Yoga and Sri Sri Ravishankar's Art of Living." In *Gurus of Modern Yoga,* edited by Mark Singleton and Ellen Goldberg, 283–307. New York: Oxford University Press, 2013.

Wailoo, Keith. *Pain: A Political History.* Baltimore: Johns Hopkins University Press, 2015.

Walker, Harry, and Iza Kavedžija. "Values of Happiness." *HAU: Journal of Ethnographic Theory* 5, no. 3 (2015): 1–23.

Weber, Max. *The Religion of India: The Sociology of Hinduism and Buddhism.* Glencoe, IL: Free Press, 1958.

Weisz, George, and Jesse Olszynko-Gryn. "The Theory of Epidemiologic Transition: The Origins of a Citation Classic." *Journal of the History of Medicine and Allied Sciences* 65, no. 3 (2010): 287–326.

Wenger, M. A., B. K. Bagchi, and B. K. Anand. "Experiments in India on 'Voluntary' Control of the Heart and Pulse." *Circulation* 24, no. 6 (1961): 1319–25.

Wigmore, Tim, Vijaya Gottumukkala, and Bernhard Riedel. "Making the Case for the Subspecialty of Onco-Anesthesia." *International Anesthesiology Clinics* 54, no. 4 (2016): 19–28.

Williams, Linda. "Melodrama Revised." In *Refiguring American Film Genres: History and Theory*, edited by Nick Browne, 42–88. Berkeley: University of California Press, 1998.

Wood, Kate, and Helen Lambert. "Coded Talk, Scripted Omissions." *Medical Anthropology Quarterly* 22, no. 3 (2008): 213–33.

Wool, Zoë H. *After War: The Weight of Life at Walter Reed*. Durham, NC: Duke University Press, 2015.

Wool, Zoë H. "In-Durable Sociality: Precarious Life in Common and the Temporal Boundaries of the Social." *Social Text* 35, no. 1 (130) (2017): 79–99.

Wool, Zoë H., and Julie Livingston. "Collateral Afterworlds." *Social Text* 35, no. 1 (130) (2017): 1–15.

Woolf, Virginia. *On Being Ill*. Paris: Paris Press, 2001.

World Health Organization. "Global Cancer Rates Could Increase by 50% to 15 Million by 2020." 2003. https://www.who.int/mediacentre/news/releases/2003/pr27/en/.

Yeager, Alyssa, Anna W. LaVigne, Ambika Rajvanshi, Birbal Mahato, Ravinder Mohan, Reena Sharma, and Surbhi Grover. "Cansupport: A Model for Home-Based Palliative Care Delivery in India." *Annals of Palliative Medicine* 5, no. 3 (2016): 166–71.

INDEX

72–74; estrangement, 67–68; lack of support, 77–78
Conway, Kathlyn, 129–30

Das, Veena, 7, 48, 71, 81–82, 203n5
denial: and concealment of cancer, 8–9, 37, 47; contexts and effects, 61–62; and distress, 61; *versus* hope, 42; in memoirs, 127
developmentalist tropes, 21
diagnoses: and concealment, 6–9; in India, 3–9, 183n11; late, 90; methods, 93–95; and social relations, 3–5
Dil Ek Mandir (film): cast, 143; irresolution in, 169; plot summary, 144–45; and the postcolonial state, 145, 147, 149; and the Ramayana, 143–45; sacrifice in, 145, 147, 149, 151–53; stills, *144, 146*
disclosure. *See* medical disclosure and nondisclosure
doubt: and cancer pain, 9, 14, 33, 111; and endurance, 5; in film, 170; *shak*, 1–3; and social relations, 4–5, 9, 33–34, 141, 171, 176
Dr. Nigam: and the author, 92–93; cancer concealment experiences, 35–36; career of, 91–92; colleague admiration for, 115; international awards, 92; on morphine use, 108; palliative care unit, 91–92, 113, 120; and patient death, 115–16; phantom limb pain patient, 106–12; poverty research, 106; prognostication abilities, 115–16; spiritual questionnaire research, 100–101; and the WHO, 92
drugs: control policies, 53, 108–9; leukemia, 44–45; morphine, 53, 66, 107–9, 199n49; opioids, 12, 107–8; Spasmolin, 72
duress, 24, 69, 88, 171, 174, 178, 180. *See also* endurance

early detection, 22
Ecks, Stefan, 44–45
empathy, 14, 86, 90–91, 111, 119–20
endemics, 174
endurance, 171–81, 204n11
epidemiological transition theory, 20, 188n67
ethics: in aesthetic representations, 121; of concealment, 8–9, 47, 61–62, 183n11; and diagnoses under precarity, 4–5; disclo-

sure and nondisclosure, 8; of endurance, 173–75, 178–80; of ordinary realism, 173; palliative care research, 104, 198n42

film: affluence in, 160–63; Amitabh Bachchan in, 153, 155, 161, 163; *Anand*, 25, 153–55, 161, 165, 202n15; *Ankhiyon Ke Jharokhon Se*, 156–58, 163; and author's ethnography, 143, 156; concealment and disclosure, 156, 158–60, 162, 168; criticism of, 142, 168; *Dard Ka Rishta*, 164–68; and the Dutt family, 163–65, 167; endurance in, 179–80; historical changes in, 155–56, 163, 167–68; irresolution in, 169–70; magical patient trope, 154–55, 160–61; melodrama in, 151–53, 167–69; *Milli*, 155, 161; *Munna Bhai M.B.B.S.*, 167–68; mythological references, 143–45, 149; optimism themes, 154–55; pathos in, 142–43, 152, 168; patient deaths, 142; and the postcolonial state, 145, 147, 149, 153, 155; *Prem Geet*, 158–60; reality in, 163–68; restitution themes, 155; *Saathi*, 147–49, 151–52, 169; sacrifices, 151–52, 155–56, 158, 167; *Satyakam*, 149–53, 169; social messages in, 163, 170; spreading fear, 142; themes of, 143; *Vaada Raha*, 160–61, 163; *Waqt: The Race against Time*, 161; women in, 152–53, 159–60, 169. *See also Dil Ek Mandir*
film, men's sacrifices in: to country, 169; *Dil Ek Mandir*, 145, 147, 149, 151–52; and family, 152, 158; low-stakes, 162; *Saathi*, 149, 151–52; to vocation, 145, 149, 158, 163, 168
film, women's sacrifices in: denials of, 159–60; *Dil Ek Mandir*, 145, 147, 152–53; as durative, 152–53, 168–69; male imposition of, 169; *Saathi*, 149, 152–53
Fischer, Michael, 81
Foucault, Michel, 174
François, Anne-Lise, 9
Frank, Arthur, 129

Ganti, Tejaswini, 143
Geertz, Clifford, 189n85
Gleevec, 44–45
the global south, 9–12, 16, 85
Good, Byron J., 7–8, 41–42

metaphors, 26, 55–56, 189n88
methodology, author's, 28
Moran-Thomas, Amy, 10–11, 186n35
morphine, 53, 66, 107–9, 199n49
mythology, 80–83, 143–45, 149

Nargis, 163–65
National Cancer Control Program, 22, 45
National Institute of Cancer Prevention and
    Research, 22–23
Nehru, Jawaharlal, 86, 196n11
new religious movements, 101–2
noncommunicable diseases (NCDs), 15–16,
    21, 105
nondisclosure. See concealment of cancer;
    medical disclosure and nondisclosure
non-governmental organizations (NGOs), 30,
    53, 177. See also Cansupport

opioids, 12, 107–8. See also morphine
optimism: cruel, 128–29; in film, 154–55; in
    memoirs, 125, 128–29, 179; rejections of,
    173; and suffering, 172–73. See also hope

pain: empathizing with, 111; and endurance,
    176–78; and endurance ethics, 176–77;
    epidemics, in lower- and middle-income
    countries, 12; gate-control theory, 111;
    versus hope, 10; neuromatrix model, 14,
    111; and physician-patient relationship, 14;
    and psychological experiences, 111, 176;
    research on, 111
pain, cancer: American diagnostic instru-
    ments, 96; assessment questionnaires,
    92–96; and bodily discourses, 13; and
    center-periphery relationships, 10; commu-
    nicating, 14; constancy of, 176; and death,
    12; and doubt, 9, 14, 33, 111; drug prescrip-
    tions, 108; as epidemic, 12; expert knowl-
    edge, 13–14; in the global south, 10–12;
    hope discourses, 11–12; inevitability of, 90;
    Lancet Commission report on, 90, 197n16;
    and late diagnoses, 90; limiting sociality,
    9; management strategies, 11–12; and na-
    tional development, 90; and new religious
    movements, 102; opioid restrictions, 12,
    107–8; palliative care, 9–10, 13; psychoso-

cial model, 14, 33, 93, 99, 105, 120, 176; and
    social relations, 5, 176; spirituality and yoga
    research, 13, 95–106, 199n44; and survival-
    oriented events, 11; technical knowledge of,
    13–14; total concept, 85; treatment as care,
    11; treatment attitudes, 11–12; and treatment
    inaccessibility, 10; treatment in the global
    south, 9–12; ubiquity of, 90; undertreat-
    ment of, 11. See also palliative care
palliative care, 9–10; Cansupport model, 52;
    delivery models debate, 50–52; Distress In-
    ventory of Cancer, 93; and empathy, 90–91,
    111, 176; in the global south, 85; hospital
    units, 84–85; Kerala Neighborhood Net-
    work model, 51–53; and malpractice suspi-
    cions, 118–19; morphine addiction claims,
    108–9; patient symptoms, 115; practice
    versus research, 119–20; specialists in, 12,
    50; and structural failures, 120. See also All
    India Institute of Medical Sciences, pallia-
    tive care unit
palliative care research: at AIIMS, 92–94; and
    asceticism research, 97–98; ethical prob-
    lems, 104, 198n42; versus practice, 119–20;
    spirituality, 13, 95–102, 105–6, 119; yoga's
    effects, 102–5, 199n44
Pinto, Sarah, 8, 48, 60, 80–81, 85
postcolonial state, 19–20, 145, 147, 149, 153,
    155, 187n64
Povinelli, Elizabeth, 25, 204n9
psychosocial pain model, 14, 33, 93, 98–99,
    105, 120, 176
public health catastrophe narratives, 16, 186n36

Rapp, Rayna, 179
Remembrance Day, 54–61, 63
Robbins, Joel, 171–72
ruins, 88, 196n11

sacrifice: and conjugality, 74; in film, 151–52,
    155–56, 158, 167; in memoirs, 134, 136. See
    also film, men's sacrifices in; film, women's
    sacrifices in
Sameera (medical resident), 1–2
Saria, Vaibhav, 50
Scarry, Elaine, 9, 199n51
secrecy and intimacy, 41

INDEX 223

www.ingramcontent.com/pod-product-compliance
Lightning Source LLC
Chambersburg PA
CBHW050352270326
41926CB00016B/3713